Hand Book of
Health Education
and Community
Pharmacy

Hand Book of
Health Education and Community Pharmacy

For First Year Diploma in Pharmacy & B. Pharm.

(According to new syllabus as prescribed by P.C.I. in education regulation 1991, implemented in the year 1993).

ASHOK K. GUPTA
M.Pharm. (Pharmaceutics)
Head of Department, Pharmacy
Govt. Polytechnic for Women, Chandigarh

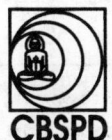

CBSPD

CBS Publishers & Distributors Pvt Ltd

New Delhi • Bengaluru • Chennai • Kochi • Kolkata • Lucknow • Mumbai
Hyderabad • Jharkhand • Nagpur • Patna • Pune • Uttarakhand

Hand Book of
Health Education
and Community
Pharmacy

ISBN: 978-81-239-0424-5

Published by Satish Kumar Jain and Produced by Varun Jain for

CBS Publishers & Distributors Pvt Ltd

4819/XI Prahlad Street, 24 Ansari Road, Daryaganj, New Delhi 110 002, India. 4819/XI Prahlad Street, 24 Ansari Road, Daryaganj, New Delhi 110 002, India.
Ph: 23289259, 23266861   Website: www.cbspd.com
                                 e-mail: delhi@cbspd.com
Corporate Office: 204 FIE, Industrial Area, Patparganj, Delhi 110 092
Ph: 011-4934 4934   Fax: 011-4934 4935   e-mail: publishing@cbspd.com;
                                             publicity@cbspd.com

Branches

- **Bengaluru:** Seema House 2975, 17th Cross, K.R. Road, Banasankari 2nd Stage, Bengaluru 560 070, Karnataka
  Ph: +91-80-26771678/79   Fax: +91-80-26771680   e-mail: bangalore@cbspd.com
- **Chennai:** 7, Subbaraya Street, Shenoy Nagar, Chennai 600 030, Tamil Nadu, India
  Ph: +91-44-26680620/26681266   Fax: +91-44-42032115   e-mail: chennai@cbspd.com
- **Kochi:** 42/1325, 1326, Power House Road, Opp KSEB, Power House, Ernakulam 682 018, Kochi, Kerala, India
  Ph: +91-484-4059061-65, 67   Fax: +91-484-4059065   e-mail: kochi@cbspd.com
- **Kolkata:** 147, Hind Ceramics Compound, 1st Floor, Nilgunj Road, Belghoria, Kolkata-700056, West Bengal, India
  Ph: +033-25633055, 033-25633056   e-mail: kolkata@cbspd.com
- **Lucknow:** Basement, Khushnuma Complex, 7 Meerabai Marg (Behind Jawahar Bhawan), Lucknow-226001, UP, India
  Ph: +91-522-4000032   e-mail: tiwari.lucknow@cbspd.com
- **Mumbai:** PWD Shed, Gala no 25/26, Ramchandra Bhatt Marg, Next to JJ Hospital Gate no. 2, Opp. Union Bank of India Noorbaug, Mumbai-400009, Maharashtra, India
  Ph: 022-66661880/89   e-mail: mumbai@cbspd.com

Representatives

• Hyderabad	0-9885175004	• Jharkhand	0-9811541605	• Nagpur	0-8692091830
• Patna	0-9334159340	• Pune	0-9664372571	• Uttarakhand	0-9716462459

Printed at: Neekunj Print Process, Sonepat, Haryana, India

SYLLABUS

THEORY (50 HOURS)

1. **Concept of Health :** Definitions of physical health, mental health, social health, spiritual health, determinants of health, indicators of health, concept of disease, natural history of diseases, the disease agents, concept of prevention of diseases.

2. **Nutrition and Health :** Classification of foods, requirements, diseases induced due to deficiency of proteins, vitamins and minerals – treatment and prevention.

3. **Demography and Family Planning:** Demography cycle, fertility, family planning, contraceptive methods, behavioural methods, natural family planning method, chemical method, mechanical methods, hormonal contraceptives, population problem of India.

4. **First Aid :** Emergency treatment in shock, snake-bite, burns, poisoning, heart of disease, fractures and resuscitation methods. Elements of minor surgery and dressings.

5. **Environment and Health :** Sources of water supply, water pollution, purification of water, health and air, noise, light, solid waste disposal and control, medical entomology, arthropod borne diseases and their control, rodents, animals and diseases.

6. **Fundamental Principles of Microbiology :** Classification of microbes, isolation, staining techniques of organisms of common diseases.

7. **Communicable Diseases :** Causative agents, mode of transmission and prevention.

    (a) *Respiratory infections* – Chicken pox, Measles, Influenza, Diphtheria, Whooping cough and Tuberculosis.

    (b) *Intestinal infections* – Poliomyelitis, Hepatitis, Cholera, Typhoid, food poisoning, Hookworm infection.

    (c) *Arthropod borne infections* – Plague, Malaria, Filariasis.

    (d) *Surface infections* – Rabies, Trachoma, Tetanus, Leprosy.

    (e) *Sexually transmitted diseases* – Syphilis, Gonorrhoea, AIDS.

8. **Non-communicable Diseases :** Causative agents, prevention, care and control. Cancer, Diabetes, Blindness, Cardiovascular diseases.

9. **Epidemiology :** Its scope, methods, uses; dynamics of diseases transmission. Immunity and immunisation; Immunological products and their dose schedule. Principles of disease control and prevention, hospital acquired infection, prevention and control. Disinfection, types of disinfection, disinfection procedures for faeces, urine, sputum, room, linen, dead bodies, instruments.

PREFACE

According to the slogan 'Health for all' by the year 2000, the Government of India is committed to provide physical, mental and social health to its citizens by the year 2000. For attaining this goal the doctors, nurses, pharmacists and all other persons engaged in the health care of the community are involved for the purpose. In this context the pharmacist has to play a great role in the implementation of National Programmes regarding health education because he is in direct contect with the public. The Govt. of India has recognised the pharmacist as an important member of health team who can act as a health counseller in rural as well as urban areas.

In recent years the course contents of Diploma in Pharmacy have been revised accordingly and an independent subject of health education and community pharmacy have been introduced.

Keeping in view the needs of teachers, students and community pharmacists the author has ventured to write the present book namely Hand Book of Health Education and Community Pharmacy so as to provide the subject matter in a precise and simple language supported by suitable diagrams wherever necessary.

I am sure this book will be warmly accepted by the teachers and students of pharmacy which will create interest in the subject.

The readers are requested to provide necessary feed back information for further improvement of the book which will be duly acknowledged.

My sincere thanks are due to Shri S.S. Bajaj, Head, Department of Pharmacy Govt. Polytechnic for Women, Chandigarh who has been a guiding spirit in this work.

I am grateful to my colleagues, teachers and students who have encouraged and inspired me to write this book.

My thanks are due to Shri Satish Jain and Shri Vinod Jain of CBS Publishers & Distributors who have brought out this book in a short span of time in spite of heavy seasonal work.

October 1995   **Ashok K. Gupta**

CONTENTS

1

CONCEPT OF HEALTH

The various terms used in relation to health are discussed below :

1. HYGIENE

The word 'hygiene' is derived from the Greek word Hygeia – the Goddess of health who looks after the health of people. The word hygeine has been defined in a number of ways, (i) Hygiene is the science and art of preserving and improving health, (ii) Hygiene is the science of health and embraces all factors which contribute to healthful living by preventing disease either in the individual or in the community. When the different measures are applied for the well being of the community as a whole in an organised manner, it is known as public health or community hygiene.

Personal hygiene is the term used for improvement of hygiene of an individual or a person like care of skin, hair, teeth, eyes, ear, hands, feet and private parts. Social hygiene is usually the term used for dealing with problems or sex especially for control of venereal diseases.

2. HEALTH

The term health has been defined in a number of ways but there is no agreed definition of health. For a lay man the term health means a person having a sound mind, in a sound body in a sound family and in a sound environment. According to World Health Organisation (WHO) the term health is defined as "Health is a state of complete physical, mental and social well-being and not merely absence of disease or infirmity."

Perfect health, optimum health or positive health has three constituents i.e. physical health, mental health and spiritual health. Along with these three constituents fourth one i.e. financial health is also very important. If the financial health remains poor it affects the rest of the three constituents. In other ways it is the controller of all the constituents of perfect health, pleasure and peace of life. Positive health means to promote and maintain health whereas negative health means scientific efforts for prevention and cure of diseases.

The important factors for promoting and maintaining good health include :

1. Supply of fresh air, light and potable water.
2. Balanced diet.
3. Proper healthful shelter.
4. Adequate clothing.
5. Hygienic environmental sanitation.
6. Protection from communicable and non-communicable diseases.
7. Adequate physical activity, rest and relaxation according to individual needs.
8. Suitable occupation with job satisfaction.
9. Good and simple habits with leisure and pleasure.

All these factors help to maintain a normal balance of body which is must for positive health. The study of all these factors is known as preventive and social medicine. If any of the above factors is not available then there are chances of illness leading to negative health.

3. PREVENTIVE AND SOCIAL MEDICINE

The terms hygiene and public health have been replaced by preventive and social medicine or social and preventive medicine. Since now-a-days air, water, food and surroundings are polluted, a man has to live and adjust in the conditions of pollution and how far and to want extent he will be able to develop immunity against every sort of pollution is a question mark. Infections are increasing day by day due to pollution, contamination, adulteration and environmental insanitation.

'Prevention is better than cure' is an old proverb but now a days a great importance is being given to this proverb. A man is a social being. Daily he comes in contact with neighbours, friends, domestic animals and pets. For basic necessities of life he depends on air, water and food which all are polluted and are sources of diseases. Similarly he comes in contact with many kinds of micro-organisms which are freely present in air and water which lead to spreading of diseases. Therefore preventive measures must be taken to prevent the spread of diseases. This can best be achieved by adopting good habits of cleanliness of individuals and surrounding, using clean water, living in well ventilated and clean rooms, keeping healthy domestic animals and pets and taking medicines for preventing diseases, as in the case of malaria or eye flu epidemic one should take proper medicines or precautions as a preventive measure. Vaccination must be got done to prevent the spread of diseases. Preventive medicine does not only include vaccine and sera but also include the role of vitamins, minerals, proteins, carbohydrates and fats in the balanced diet.

Social medicine : Social medicine is now taking the place of public health.The content of social medicine consists of aspects of health, happiness and efficiency. Its aim includes intensive study of environmental and other factors such as condition of work, home, background, nutrition and social adjustments which cause diseases and application of that study for the benefit of man so as to prevent diseases and promote good health.

Social medicine is the science and is connected with the community health in respect of social, economic and environmental conditions.

Different authors have expressed social medicine in different names. Professor Winslow defined it as an art of prolonging life and promoting physical and mental health through organised community efforts for the sanitation and environmental control of community infection and also the social machinery which ensures every individual a standard of living, adequate for the maintenance of health.

Diseases can be comparatively easily prevented rather than cured if the basic conditions and cause of the disease is identified. Social and preventive medicine help to prevent the diseases to a great extent. Sanitary and hygienic conditions will help in the prevention of diseases but will not gurantee for total prevention of disease because there are so many other factors such as social, psychological and economical which influence the health of a person. Undesirable habits, traditions and conditions of living can be equally responsible for the sufferings of an individual and ultimately community as a whole. Illiteracy, poverty, unemployment, under-employment and economic tensions are other causes of ill health.

Population of the world is increasing fast and with the increase in population the cases of communicable, non-communicable and venereal diseases are also increasing which can be prevented with the help of social and preventive medicine.

Thus the health of the people depends primarily on the social, economic and environmental conditions under which they live and work. Health of a person also depends on water, food, physical surroundings, occupation and standard of living. Underlying all these conditions the main problems of ill health include poverty, illiteracy, family size, malnutrition, poor housing, deep-rooted customs and habits.

Since these are the days of anxiety, worry and tension therefore real happiness and sound health is difficult to achieve. Hence all people are suffering from either physical, mental, social or spiritual health. In rural areas the subject of social and preventive medicine is of great importance due to bad hygienic environmental sanitation. Many diseases can be easily prevented by adopting suitable preventive measures.

4. COMMUNITY HEALTH/COMMUNITY MEDICINE

The terms community health and/or community medicine are being used in an interchangeable manner. The term community health is more commonly used by the health workers and has gained wide acceptance as the overall emphasis is on health in all community programmes. The term community health is of recent origin and merely replaces the previous terms hygiene and public health or preventive and social medicine.

According to World Health Organisation Expert Committee on community health nursing the community health is defined as a system of delivery of comprehensive health care to the people by a team of medical persons to improve the health of community. Community health or community medicine programmes include preventive and social medicine along with curative and health promotion services in an attempt to promote a state of positive health in the community. In fact, the health of whole of the community depends on personal habits of various individuals who constitute the community. So, dirty or unhygienic habits of individual persons can create problems for whole of the community. For example a person may be perfectly healthy by adoping various means of livelihood like taking balanced diet, having clean personal habits and living in neat, clean and well-ventilated house etc. But if the other people living in his neighbourhood dump garbage in open space where flies, mosquitoes and other disease producing germs will grow and spoil the neat and clean surroundings. This will ultimately lead to diseases in the healthy person living nearby. This is one example of unhygienic conditions. Similarly a large number of other examples can be given.

The Community Health Services which are provided by the government through municipal committees or municipal corporations in cities and by panchayats in villages should cover all the fields of preventive and curative aspects like control of communicable diseases, maternal and child health services, school health services, environmental sanitation, nutrition, providing clean drinking water, good sewage disposal system, open spaces in the form of gardens, parks and play grounds. It should also include health education, family planning, social security and medical statistics.

All the above mentioned conditions are necessary for providing and maintaining good health to the whole of the community. So for the general welfare of the community we have to fight with the problems of population, poverty, unemployment, illiteracy and ill health.

Health for All

In september 1978 an international conference on primary health care was held at Alma-Ata, U.S.S.R. which issued a declaration stating that primary health care is the key to attaining "Health for all by the year 2000". The member states of W.H.O. agreed and were quick to respond to the call.

'Health for all' does not mean that in the year 2000 doctors and nurses will provide medical care to everybody in the world for all their existing ailments nor does it mean that in the year 2000 there won't be any disease, sick or disabled person. But health for all by the year 2000 means that :

1. Health care will be provided at home, school and in factories.
2. People will use better measures for preventing unavoidable illness and disability.
3. Essential health care will be provided to all individuals, families and communities in an acceptable and affordable way.
4. There will be equal distribution of all the available health resources among the population.

ASPECTS OF HEALTH
(COMPONENTS OF HEALTH)

1. PHYSICAL HEALTH

Physical health means that an individual should be physically fit. The body organs are structurally (anatomical point of view) and functionally (physiology point of view) in a normal state and there is perfect co-ordination between the organs and systems that the body as a whole functions in perfect harmony.

When a person is sick and suffering from a disease, he does not feel like eating anything, he gets weak, he does not want to talk and gets irritated even on minor matters, he does not take interest in wordly affairs, he feels depressed and miserable and his working capacity decreases.

Absence from sickness or disease does not mean that a person is healthy. Apart from sickness and disease, a healthy person should not have any physical handicap i.e. there should not be crippled arms or legs or damaged or defective eyes.

Physical health is an important component of total health. It includes hygiene of different parts of the body such as skin, hair, teeth, eyes, ears, hands, feet, rest and sleep, exercise and recreation.

Thus physical health means that an individual should be free from sickness and disease including communicable and non-communicable diseases and there should not be any deformity of the body like crippling of the limbs or damaged eyes.

2. MENTAL HEALTH

These are the days of anxiety, worry and tension and the problem of mental illness is increasing day by day not only in India but throughout the world specially in developed countries rather than developing countries. In U.S.A. nearly half of the beds in hospitals are occupied by mental patients. This is because of so called fastness in life, materialism, discontentment and restlessness. The man, today has become lonely in a crowd with degradation of human values, loss of social ties, self centred life, lack of opportunities, deprivation and increase in the expectations due to excessive use of mass media. Man has become so instrumental and self centred that he has forgotten loving each other. With the advance-ment of knowledge and skills gained about modern machanisation the man has reduced himself to a negligible part of the total machinery.

According to modern concept of W.H.O. the health is defined as the complete physical, mental and social well-being and not merely an absence of disease. Mental health is an important component of total health. As there is a saying that healthy mind resides in healthy body, physical health and mental health are interrelated with each other. If a person is physically healthy he will also become mentally healthy because the mental health depends on physical health and vice versa. Therefore good physical health is the first stepping stone to mental health. Mental health is important for an individual to enable him to lead a happy, contented and healthy social life, and to withstand the stress and strains of life in a satisfactory manner.

Mental health is defined as the ability of the individual to make personal and social adjustments. These adjustments are concerned with one's daily life in relation to others, at home and at work and he adjusts in a way acceptable to the society.

Characteristics of a Mentally Healthy Person

A Mentally Health Person has the following Characteristics :

1. A mentally healthy person feels contented, satisfied, happy, calm and cheerful. He does not condemn himself and there are no conflicts within himself. He has self repect. He neither underestimates nor over-estimates his own ability.

2. A mentally healthy person is able to think for himself and take

his own decisions. He does not shirk his responsibilities and is able to meet the demands of life.

3. He has firm determination and self control. He faces problems and tries to solve them intelligently. He is not dominated by fear, anger, love, jealousy, stress and worries.

4. A mentally healthy person is able to adjust with other people, make sincere and long-lasting friends and does not feel isolated. He understands problems and emotional needs of others and tries to be considerate and courteous in his dealings with others. He accepts criticism and does not get easily upset and tries to overcome emotions.

5. A mentally healthy person adjusts himself successfully to the changing situations and does not get upset when things go wrong, whereas some people react sharply, lose their temper, talk loudly and make everybody around uncomfortable.

Factors Leading to Mental Ill Health

1. **Heredity :** It is well known that certain mental diseases (e.g. schizophrenia) runs in families.

2. **Physical Health :** Sickness and/or disability affect mental health.

3. **Social Factors :** Worries, anxieties, emotional stress, tension, frustration, unhappy marriages, broken homes, poverty, cruelty, neglect etc. all lead to mental illness.

4. The use of alcohol and other narcotics is one of the major causes of mental ill health and has ruined many homes.

5. Irritability over trifles, fluctuation of mood, insomnia, depression, disturbed state of mind, state of fear and feeling of various non-existing complaints also lead to mental ill health.

Types of Mental Illness

Mental diseases may be divided into two groups :

(i) **Major Mental Disorders**
   (a) Schizophrenia
   (b) Manic depressive psychosis
   (c) Paronia

(ii) **Minor Mental Disorders**
   (a) Neurosis

(b) Personality disorders.

(a) Schizophrenia is a severe mental disorder (or group of disorders) characterised by disturbances in thinking, mood, perception and, at times, of posture. The patient lives in a dream world of his own.

(b) Manic depressive psychosis is a severe mental illness causing repeated episodes of extreme depression, excitement or both. These episodes can be precipitated by upsetting events but are out of proportion to these causes.

(c) Paronia is a severe mental disorder which is associated with extreme suspicion and the patient lives in a world of delusion (on irrationally held belief that cannot be altered by rational arguments. In mental illness it is often a false belief that the individual is persecuted (punished, maltreated or treated cruelly) by others.

(d) Neurosis is a mental illness in which insight is retained but there is a maladaptive way of behaving or thinking that causes suffering. The patient shows peculiar symptoms such as unwanted fears, compulsions and obsessions (fear, a fixed or false idea; continually distress).

(e) Personality disorder is the habit or tendencies and maladjusted pattern of behaviour, persisting through many years. The abnormality of behaviour must be sufficiently severe that it causes suffering either to the patient or to other people (or to both).

Warning Signs of Mental Ill Health

With the help of following questions one can gauge his own mental health. If the answer to any question is 'yes' then remedial measures should be taken so as to have good mental health.

1. Are you always worrying ?
2. Are you continuously unhappy without any reasonable causes ?
3. Do you loose your temper easily on trifles ?
4. Are you suffering from insomnia ?
5. Are you unable to concentrate on your routine work without any justifiable reason ?
6. Are you afraid without real cause ?
7. Do you dislike the company of people ?

8. Are you always right and the other person always wrong ?

9. Do you have superiority or inferiority complex ?

10. Do you remain always irritated ?

11. Do your children constantly trouble you due to any reasons ?

12. Do you get upset if the routine of your life is disturbed ?

13. Is there any quarrel among members of the family ?

14. Do you have wide fluctuations in your moods i.e. from depression to elation and back to depression ?

15. Are you suffering from various aches and pains without any diagnostic physical cause ?

Suggestions for Preventing Mental Ill Health

(i) Malnutrition which is wide spread among poor people and rural area is one of the major causes of mental retardation in children and late pregnancy which permanently affects the development of the child. Hence people should be educated regarding nutrition, health and psychosexual behaviour.

(ii) First five years of age are very important for a child because during these five years behaviour disorders commonly develop. Therefore it is very important that proper atmosphere should be provided for normal personality development of the child.

(iii) School provides a number of new experiences to the child including exposure to group life, social and academic relations. They all lead to emotional repercussions on the mind of the child. Hence better relationship between teachers and students should be developed.

(iv) Special schools should be started for providing proper guidance to the mentally retarded children.

(v) During pregnancy females should be provided special care because during this period she will be under great stress and strain due to labour pains and other obstetrical troubles. She may be emotionally disturbed :

   (a) about her capacity for bearing, delivering and nourishing the child,

   (b) about her sexual anatomy and attractiveness, and

(c) about her relation with her husband during pregnancy and the period to follow it.

(vi) Adolescent age is very crucial from mental health point of view because during this period lot of changes take place in body, sex, behaviour and personality. Youth has a tendency not to accept the ways in which their parents or seniors expect them to behave, and had a tendency to manage their own affairs themselves. This tendency leads to protest, unrest, sex and drugs etc. They are exposed to mass media which aggravate on their desires and expectations and if not fulfilled lead to frustrations. They are also exploited by politicians. Students in our country are overburdened with studies because of faulty examination system which lead to depression and frustrations.

(vii) Youth welfare programmes, social welfare programmes, opportunities for creative work, recreational facilities, happy family and social life all play an important role in maintaining and promoting normal mental health.

(viii) In old age so many problems arise regarding health and family affairs so proper medical facilities, old age homes and rehabilitation centers should be provided.

3. SOCIAL HEALTH

Man is a social animal, he cannot live individually, he will have to depend on each other to fulfil his basic necessities. In the primitive age he used to live singly and in the primitive society of tribal era. But now he is not merely a member of a family but a member of a locality, society, a city, a country or the world. The problem of an individual is considered as the problem of the area, city, country or even of the world. Therefore necessity arose for creating world organisations like World Health Organisation, United Nations Organisation, Agriculture Organisation etc. Similarly on these patterns local, district, state and national organisations are formed.

The health of the people depends primarily on the social and environmental conditions under which they live and work. Undesirable habits, traditions and living coditions are equally responsible for the sufferings of an individual and community as a whole. Economic tensions, poverty, illiteracy, unemployment and adverse social relations greatly affect the health of an individual.

In our country there are certain customs and religious obligations which affect the social health of an individual as well as community and country as a whole. For example child bearing, specially male child bearing, is a religious custom which leads to enlargement of the family and rapid increase in population. In such cases social factors and community action can play a great role in eradication of such customs.

4. SPIRITUAL HEALTH

Spiritual health is concerned with spirit or soul and is that health which evokes the good spirits and right things and keeps away from bad activities. The body is always guided by soul, if the spiritual health is sound the bad thinking is always controlled by inner soul and the person hesitates to do bad events but when the inner soul is overpowered by the mind then inner voice does not come to guide the mind thus he does not hesitate to indulge in bad activities, though he may realise his follies afterwards.

All religions are concerned mainly about the spiritual welfare. It is the supernatural power that contributes to the health of an individual. For the wellbeing of an individual in addition to physical, mental, social and spiritual components of health it is necessary to follow set rules and regulations in daily life e.g. as per saying early to bed and early to rise makes a man healthy, wealthy and wise. To do prayers in the morning and evening are healthy signs of spiritual health. Now the research has proved that the spiritual link between soul, mind and body is important in the human cure. Further studies have shown that changes in the life style of an individual can reduce the chances of diseases.

The modern system of medicine give quick cure to many diseases but do not care for the satisfaction of the patient. There should be some system that should give physical, mental as well as spiritual relief. Yoga and exercise help to a great extent in these respects.

Determinants of Health (Deciding Agents/Factors of Health)

Now a days health has become a complex issue. While studying determinants of health, all its aspects viz. physical, mental, social and spiritual must be borne in mind. All those factors that affect the various aspects of health should be considered as determinants of health. Determinants of health depend on :

(A) **Individual Factors :** An individual is responsible for his health. Even his surroundings, his habits, his way of living, the society in which he lives, the environment, his family background, his economic condition etc. all affect the health of a person. Following are the individual factors which affect health of a person :

   (i) Heredity

   (ii) Life style

(B) **Environmental or Surrounding Factors :**

   (i) Socio-economic factors

   (ii) Political will

   (iii) Availability of health services

(C) **Other Factors**

(A) INDIVIDUAL FACTORS

(i) **Heredity :** The state of health of an individual depends on genetic characters received from parents. Genes play a very important role in the health and development of a child. Many diseases are heredity e.g. haemophilia and sickle cell anaemia. Haemophilia is disease in which the blood of the patient clots very slowly due to deficiency of one of the coagulating factors. Sickle cell anaemia is a hereditary disease in which the red blood corpuscles become sickle shaped due to a defective type of haemoglobin, and their oxygen carrying capacity is greatly reduced. They ultimately lead to anaemia. Another simple example is that if parents are suffering from diabetes, their children may also suffer from diabetes.

(ii) **Life Style :** Life style of an individual plays a great role in health. It may affect health in both ways i.e. it may promote and maintain good health as it may adversly affect the health. Life style includes many personal activities like care of body, bathing, washing, care of teeth, hair, nails, posture and habits which include food, exercise, sleep, use of alcohol, narcotics and drugs. An individual learns lifestyls from his personal experiences or from others' experiences. If a person is having good habits, has better attitude towards others and has positive attitude towards life then he will enjoy physical, mental, social and spiritual health but on the other hand if a person has bad habits, he quarrels with others, indulges in the use of alcohol, narcotics or other drugs then he will not only be a problem for himself but will also affect the health of whole family, society and community.

(B) ENVIRONMENTAL OR SURROUNDING FACTORS

(i) Socio-Economic Factors

The health of an individual depends on the socio-economic factors which are governed by set rules and regulations framed and accepted by the society in which he lives. Certain customs of a particular community or society are good for healthy living but there are certain customs which are detrimental to health e.g. to serve wine on social functions. Dowry system which is a curse greatly affects health of an individual or family directly or indirectly.

The development of any society depends on the socio-economic factors of individuals. If they are financially sound there will be all round development in education, housing, social relations and hygienic conditions. With all these developments there will be improvement in standard of living which will affect the health status of an individual in many ways. Poverty is the root cause of most of the problems. Poor nutrition, illiteracy, slums, lack of basic needs, unhygienic conditions all lead to ill health. The development should not be limited to the satisfaction of basic needs only but it should go much further than that. Apart from the satisfactory provision of basic needs there should be provision for proper hygienic conditions, sewer system, *pacca* roads, well built houses, educational and recreational facilities. From all these facilities there will be development of all individuals, communities and societies which will overall affect the development of the country, thus the health of all its subjects will be affected to a great extent. Hence health and development are closely related to each other.

Financial health is the controller of all the ingredients of health, pleasure, peace of life and development. The financial health and physical health are dependent on each other. If an individual is physically healthy, he will do hard work to earn money and to remain physically fit he requires good nutrition for which money is needed. Thus financial health and physical health are interdependent. But physical and mental health are the most important among all aspects of health.

Role of Poverty in Health

Poverty is one of the major reasons for ill health of the people due to the following reasons :

1. Due to poverty, people are unable to buy sufficient food and if they buy food generally that is devoid of nutritive values which leads to deficiency disease and ruins the health of a person.
2. Poor people are mostly uneducated. They do not understand the value of balanced diet or the value of cheap articles from where they can get good nutrition. The lack of which leads to many diseases just because of ignorance.
3. Poor people live in slums which are unhygienic and breeding ground for disease-causing germs. They do not bother about their own cleanliness or unhygienic conditions of their surroundings.
4. Due to poverty, poor people are unable to get the best available medical treatment due to which the disease lingers on for a long time and ultimately leads to death of the patients.
5. Generally poor people are illiterate. They do not understand the harmful effects of alcohol, tobacco or other drugs. The use of these items ruins the health as well as financial condition of a person.

(ii) Political Will

As already discussed that poverty is the root cause of most of the health problems. The poor people living in slums are the easy target of diseases because they are deprived of all basic facilities like fresh water, proper food, houses, lighting system, environment, education and health facilities.

They live under unhygienic conditions therefore specially the children as well as other persons living in these slums are easily affected by diseases. They neither get preventive nor curative measures. But if political decisions are taken and policies are framed then within no time all types of facilities like fresh water, *pacca* houses, *pacca* roads, electricity, educational and medical facilities are provided free of cost or at reasonable cost which can certainly affect and promote the health status of these people living in slums. But all these issues are primarily of political nature.

(iii) Availability of Health Care Services

To be a healthy person is the fundamental right of all the individuals and communities of any country therefore it is the duty and responsiblity of all the state governments as well as central governments of all the respective countries to provide health care facilities to all its subjects, be it human beings, animals or plants etc. at affordable costs so that all their subjects are hale and hearty. World Health Organisation (W.H.O.) has set up a goal of achieving "Health for all by 2000 A.D." To achieve this goal greater emphasis is laid on primary health care facilities/services provided by the government as well as non-government organisations. It is not only the government or non-government organisations which should provide the basic health care facilities/services but all individuals at their own level must contribute to achieve this goal so as to promote preventive, curative and promotive health care. The basic facilities which should be provided for primary health care are as follows :

   (i) Adequate supply of safe drinking water.

  (ii) Adequate supply of nutritious food.

 (iii) Proper hygienic conditions and facilities for disposal of excreta and other wastes.

 (iv) Maternal and Child Health (M.C.H.) care and family planning services.

  (v) Preventive measures against diseases and immunisation against infectious diseases.

 (vi) Educating the people regarding healthy ways of living.

(vii) Provision of essential drugs preferably at doorsteps in slum areas.

(viii) Provision for adequate medical facilities.

(C) OTHER FACTORS

The other factors on which the health of an individual depends include age, sex, race, rural or urban living, health facilities, nutrition, environment etc. The natural factors include air, water, soil, climate, microorganisms, rodents, insects, plants etc.

INDICATORS OF HEALTH

Health indicators are the factors which give information and are required to assess the health of the community as well as to find out how far a given person is healthy. They are also required for comparison of health between the communities and also in the same community over certain period of time. Health indicators are also required for providing health and nursing care and for monitoring the progress of health programmes. Usually these indicators are calculated as rates for a particular base over a definite period of time like a year or so. The indicators of health are as follows :

   (i) Mortality indicators
   (ii) Morbidity indicators
   (iii) Health care services indicators

(i) Mortality Indicators (Death Rate)

Mortality rate of children of any country is the direct indicator for gauging the state of development of the country. A high mortality rate of children in a country indicates that the country is undeveloped or under-developed. But on the other hand if the mortality rate of children is low, it shows that the country is highly developed. The death rate of infants (children below one year of age) is called Infant Mortality Rate (IMR) and the death rate of children below 5 years of age is called Under Five Mortality Rate (UFMR). Infant Mortality Rate is calculated as follows:

$$\text{Infant Mortality Rate} = \frac{\text{No. of deaths registered or estimated of children below one year of age in an area}}{\text{No. of live births registered or estimated during the year in the area}} \times 1000$$

Similarly crude death rate is calculated which is a significant indicator of health. If the death rate is high, it indicates that the health of the community is poor. Crude death rate may be defined as the number of deaths per 1000 population per year in a given community.

$$\text{Death rate} = \frac{\text{No. of deaths in the year}}{\text{Mean population during the year}} \times 1000$$

Life expectancy i.e. the age upto which male or female will live is another indicator of health status of a community. A low expectation of life indicates a low level of health and high expectation of life indicates high level of health.

In our country the Child Mortality Rate and Crude Death Rate are quite large so suitable measures will have to be taken to improve the health of the community.

(ii) Morbidity Rate (Disease Rate)

The morbidity rate is the number of cases of a disease found to occur in a stated number of population, usually given as cases per 1,00,000 or per million. Annual figures for morbidity rate give the incidence of the disease, which is the number of new cases reported in the year. The morbidity indicators are used to describe the ill health of those who are actually suffering from disease or illness. It includes the statistical data showing notification of disease and number of cases admitted in the hospital.

(iii) Health Care Services Indicators

Health care services indicators are determined from doctor-population ratio, doctor-nurse ratio, population-health centre ratio, population-bed ratio etc. The indication of health status does not depend only on the availability of health care services but depends on the extent to which these services are utilized.

Besides the above mentioned indicators there are so many other indicators of health such as :

    (a) Nutritional status indicators

    (b) Sanitation indicators

    (c) Socio-economic indicators

    (d) Quality of life indicators

Advantages of Good Health

If a person is healthy his efficiency to do work will increase. By doing hard work he will earn more money thus will be financially sound and his standard of living will increase. Thus the increased efficiency of a man due to good health contributes to his own progress, the progress of the community and progress of the nation as a whole. Good health makes a man happy, cheerful and life joyful experience. According to old saying– 'Health is Wealth'. If health is lost everything is lost.

Concept of Disease

The WHO has defined health but not disease. This is because disease may occur in different varieties ranging from subclinical to severe or fatal illness which may even lead to death. The onset of disease may be sudden or prolonged as in the case of food poisoning and cancer respectively. Some diseases are short lived but others may remain for the whole life. The final outcome of the disease may be recovery, disability, illness or death of the person. Fortunately some of the diseases are recovered by itself e.g. healing of wound. This ability of healing is known as the natural healing power.

The term disease has been defined in many ways but an adequate definition of disease is yet to be found. Some of the definitions of disease are given below :

(a) Disease is an abnormal state of body when some of the organ(s) of the body is not functioning in a normal way or properly due to harmful effects of the process.

(b) Disease is "any deviation from function or complete physical or mental well-being".

(c) Ecologists define disease as an outcome of the disturbance of delicate balance between man and his environment.

(d) According to dictionary meaning disease is a disorder with a specific cause and recognisable signs and symptoms. The word disease conveys different meanings to different persons. To the patient it means disease i.e. discomfort or disharmony with his environment; to the doctor it means signs and symptoms and to a pathologist it means one or more structural changes.

Natural History of Disease

The concept of disease has changed with the passage of time i.e. from the supernatural theory to the germ theory and to the theory of multiple causes.

(a) **Supernatural Theory :** The pre-historic or premitive man believed that disease was caused due to some supernatural powers or bad spirits that inhabited animals, plants, water and air etc. Therefore in this age the treatment of diseases was based on religion, magic and tantras mantras. Though the science has advanced to a great extent but still people believe in magic and tantra mantara and some of the diseases are cured by worshipping the Almighty God.

(b) **Germ Theory :** In early 20th century with the advancement of science and study of microbiology it was put forth that the diseases are caused by micro-organisms that enter into the body of the host and not due to evil spirits or bad air. Bacteria and germs are the sole causes of diseases.

(c) **Theory of Multiple Causes :** According to this theory the diseases are caused not only due to one reason but there are a number of causes which may include social, economic, cultural, psychological and environmental. There are a number of diseases which are caused by different reasons and tuberculosis is a representative disease which is caused by multiple reasons like poverty, malnutrition, poor hygiene, poor housing, overcrowding, illiteracy etc.

The natural history of any disease has been divided into two phases i.e.

(i) prepathogenic phase and

(ii) pathogenic phase

(i) **Prepathogenic Phase :** Prepathogenic phase is the period before the onset of disease in man or before the appearance of signs and symptoms of a disease in man. The disease-producing agents of many diseases are present in the surroundings or in the environment but has not yet entered in man.

There are three factors which are necessary for producing the disease which include agent, host and environment. These three factors are known as epidemiological triad. In the absence of any one of these factors disease cannot occur. When these three factors are available and the person is susceptible and physically weak then the causative agent will enter into the body to produce a disease.

(ii) **Pathogenic Phase :** Pathogenic phase is the period when the disease-producing agent has entered into the body of the host and signs and symptoms of the disease start appearing. In certain cases the causative agent has to multiply to attain strength so as to bring physiological changes or damage the tissues. The period from the entry of causative agent into the body to the appearance of first symptoms of the disease is known as incubation period. The incubation period varies from disease to disease. After incubation period it takes some more time that clear cut signs and symptoms of the disease are produced. This period is known as pathogenesis period. During this period if proper treatment is not done it may lead to severe illness, disability of the organ involved or even death of the host.

Every disease has its own natural history and shows characteristic signs and symptoms but it is not necessary that all the individuals will have the same natural history and signs and symptoms of the disease. However by knowing the natural history of the disease one can take firm steps in the prevention, spread and treatment of the disease.

Disease Agents

It is well known fact that every disease is caused by some agent which is defined as a substance living or non-living or a force tangible or intangible the excessive presence or relatively lack of which may initiate a disease process. A disease is produced by a single agent or more than one agent independently or in combination with each other. The various disease agents are classified as follows :

(i) **Biological Agent :** These are the living agents which include bacteria, fungi, parasites, protozoa and viruses etc. These agents are found in man, animals, insects, soil and environment.

(ii) **Physical Agents :** Exposure to excessive heat, cold, pressure, radiations, humidity and electricity etc. may lead to illness.

(iii) **Chemical Agents :**

(a) Exogenic agents i.e. agents which are present outside the human body like dust, fumes, gases, metals, allergenic agents etc.

(b) Endogenic agents i.e. agents which are produced inside the body as a result of metabolic changes like urea leads to uremia, uric acid leads to gout and ketones lead to ketosis.

(iv) **Mechanical Agents :** Accidental exposure to chronic friction and other mechanical forces may lead to injuries, crushing, tearing, fracture, dislocation or death.

(v) **Nutritional Agents :** Nutritional agents include carbohydrates, proteins, fats, vitamins, minerals and water. An excess or deficiency of these agents may lead to nutritional diseases like obesity, anaemia, goitre, kwashiorkar, marasmus, night blindness, scurvy etc.

Apart from above mentioned disease agents the other factors which are responsible for disease include age, sex, race, marital status, heredity, occupation, customs and habits, life style; physical, biological and social environment etc.

Concept of Prevention of Diseases

"Prevention is better than cure". According to this saying suitable preventive measures must be taken for the occurance and spread of diseases. The factors that are hazardous to health must be taken care of. Now-a-days the concept of prevention has become broad based and is defined in terms of three levels which include :

    (a) Primary prevention

    (b) Secondary prevention

    (c) Tertiary prevention

(A) PRIMARY PREVENTION

Primary prevention may be defined as "action taken prior to the onset of disease which removes the possibility of ever occurance of a disease". The action taken mainly include all those factors which raise the standard of living of community and promote the general well being of the society. These factors can be studied under two headings i.e.

    (a) Health promotion measures

    (b) Specific protective measures

(a) Health Promotion Measures

These include :

    (i) Maintenance of a healthy environment.

    (ii) Maintenance of personal hygiene.

    (iii) Eating of adequate balanced diet

    (iv) Provision of safe water supply

(v) Provision of proper disposal of human excreta and domestic wastes.

(vi) Provision of well managed sewer system.

(vii) Isolation of infected persons.

(viii) Immunisation.

(ix) Maintenance of healthy and clean sex life.

(x) Motivation of the people to avoid the use of tobacco, alcohol and drugs.

(b) Specific Protective Measures

Specific diseases can be prevented by taking specific measures against these diseases. For example tuberculosis, diphtheria, pertusis, tetanus, polio, measles etc. can be prevented by immunisation at proper age and time. Since children are more susceptible to these diseases, so all the children should be vaccinated so as to get immunity from these diseases. In fact most of the children's diseases can be prevented by vaccination. Ricketsia and scurvy can be prevented by administration of Vitamin D and Vitamin C respectively. Similarly industrial accidents can be prevented by using specific protective devices like goggles, gloves or shields against carcinogens, allergens and occupational hazards etc.

It is worthwhile to mention that many developed countries have succeeded in eliminating most of the infectious diseases by primary prevention and efforts are being made to prevent chronic diseases by primary prevention e.g. stoppage of smoking, drinking, dietary control and physical exercise etc.

Primary prevention is less expensive, safe and more effective way of preventing diseases in comparison to secondary and tertiary preventive techniques. Nature has provided some defence mechanisms in our body which will prevent the entry of disease producing micro-organisms in the body or destroy them. These defence mechanisms include white blood cells (W.B.C.), skin hair, eye lids, eye lashes, and tears etc.

(B) SECONDARY PREVENTION

Secondary prevention may be defined as "action which halts the progress of a disease at its initial stage and prevents complications".

Although all precautions and care is taken to prevent the diseases but even then the causative factor succeeds in inducing the diseased state in the person. Now-a-days a number of vaccines have been developed to prevent various diseases but we do not have vaccines for preventing all types of diseases. For diseases like cancer, diabetes, epilepsy, leprosy, syphilis and malaria etc. there is no vaccine available. In such cases early diagnosis and treatment is the only solution. The earliest identification and diagnosis of the disease will be in the benefit of the patient as well as doctor. Earlier diagnosis will help the physician in preventing the disease with proper treatment and to control further progress of the disease.

Some of the methods by which early diagnosis or identification of the disease can be made include screening surveys, periodic examination and special examination of people who are at high risk of disease.

Secondary prevention is often more expensive and less effective than primary prevention in controlling the transmission of diseases.

(C) TERTIARY PREVENTION

If primary prevention fails the person gets disease. The early diagnosis and proper treatment helps the patient for early recovery. But in certain cases due to typical nature of the disease, it cannot be diagnosed at its early stages. Under such circumstances if the disease is not handled properly or the patient is not attended properly it may lead to various complications which may result in permanent disability or death of the patient. The aim of the tertiary prevention is to reduce further complications or permanent disability in the patient. It includes disability prevention and rehabilitation of the patient.

Permanent disability can be prevented by immunising the infants against polio, tuberculosis etc. Disability due to industrial accidents can be prevented by wearing goggles, gloves, hoods etc. Surgical operations can limit the disability to a great extent. Adequate treatment and physiotherapy alone can reduce the duration of disability.

Rehabilitation of the handicapped persons is very important which can be brought about by medical, social, educational and vocational measures. He should be rehabilitated in such a way that he does not feel ignored, earns his livlihood and becomes a useful member of the society. It can be done through physiotherapy, occupational therapy, vocational rehabilitation, sheltered workshops, colonies, selective changes in occupation, opening of hostels and schools for handicapped children and attachment of artificial limbs to an accident victim etc.

Health Education

Health education is defined as a process of imparting information about health in such a way that the people are motivated to use the information for the protection and promotion of health of individuals, their families and communities. Every community health worker, be it a doctor, nurse or pharmacist is a health educator. Our government has set up community health centres throughout the country to impart health education, vaccination facilities and to treat common diseases.

Aims and Objects of Health Education

1. Health should be realised as a valuable asset and essential for life in the community.
2. To make awareness about the skills, knowledge and attitude so that the people may solve health problems by their own actions and efforts.
3. To encourage the public to take benefit of health services for the benefit of individuals and community as a whole e.g. family planning programme etc.
4. To provide information and create awareness among the public so as to relieve them from misconceptions, doubts and ignorance.
5. To create healthy habits and change their modes of life. For example many diseases are developed by using contaminated water and by defaecating in the open. If they are imparted knowledge about harmful effects of such habits they may be relieved from many diseases.

Areas of Health Education

Health education has a very wide area of imparting knowledge to people which are described below :

1. It gives knowledge regarding structure and functions of the body and tells how to keep physically and mentally fit, about exercise, rest and sleep; harmful effects of alcohol, tobacco and drugs on the body.

2. It gives knowledge regarding various nutrients present in different food materials and making a balanced diet from available foods. It also gives knowledge regarding storage, preparation, cooking, serving and eating of food.

3. It gives information about the causes of various common diseases, how they spread and protection from these diseases. People should be encouraged to participate in the national programmes of disease control and eradication.

4. It imparts knowledge about personal and environmental hygiene. Personal hygiene includes bathing, washing, clothing, toilets, care of feet, nails, teeth, hair and skin; spitting, coughing, sneezing and developing clean habits in young children. Environmental hygiene include cleaning, proper lighting and ventilation of houses; supply of clean water, control of rats and mice; proper sewage and disposal of refuge etc.

5. It imparts knowledge about causes and protection from environmental pollution.

6. It gives knowledge about the best use of health services provided by the government or voluntary organisations.

7. Health education provides knowledge on first aid in accidental cases and handling of emergency situations like child birth.

Now a days health education has become a very important subject. The government has started community health centres where public is imparted health education. India has a very large population out of which majority is illiterate who do not know the ways and means of healthful living. A large number of people die every year because of ignorance. Therefore it becomes necessary to give knowledge to such people through health education. A few doctors, nurses, pharmacists or health workers are not sufficient to impart health education to whole of population of India. Health education can be spread easily if large number of men, women and voluntary organisations come forward who can take the message of health education to more and more people throughout the country. Such an involvement of the people in health education will lead to quick initiative in tackling urgent health problems. For example if any factory is polluting the nearby river from where the people take their water requirements for drinking, bathing and washing purposes, if the people are aware of the harmful effects

of such pollution, they can collectively force the owner of the factory
to stop this practice of polluting the river water or they may take the
help of authorities concerned in such matters.

Methods of Health Education

Health education can be imparted by following methods

A. Methods of Group Teaching
1. Lectures
2. Films and charts
3. Radio
4. T.V.
5. Flash cards
6. Cinema slides
7. Group discussions
8. Panel discussions
9. Symposium
10. Workshops
11. Demonstrations

B. Methods of Education of the General Public
1. Posters
2. Health magazines
3. Press
4. Films
5. Radio and T.V.
6. Health exhibitions
7. Health museums
8. Through katha-varta, prabhat pheries, songs and dramas etc.

2

NUTRITION AND HEALTH

Nutrition may be defined as the science of food and its relationship to health. It is one of the most importants elements of health care. Now a days greater emphasis is laid on nutrition to provide better health to the families and communities. Undernourishment and malnutrition lead to so many diseases like tuberculosis, goitre, anaemia, beri-beri, night blindness and infections of skin, gastro-intestinal and respiratory tract. The dietary factors play a major role in non-communicable diseases like heart disease, diabetes, obesity, hypertension, disorder of liver and gall bladder etc. Poverty, economic inability and illiteracy are the important causes of malnutrition. Therefore diseases are more common in poor people rather than economically better and educated people.

Through centuries food has been recognised as an important constituent for human beings in health and diseases and major time was devoted in production or search of food. Until the turn of the century the science of nutrition had a limited range and greater emphasis was laid on carbohydrates, proteins and fats but the discovery of vitamins revolutionised the science of nutrition and gained recognition as a scientific discipline.

FOOD

A food may be defined as any substance which when taken into the body can be utilized to provide heat or energy, to maintain and compensate wear and tear of tissues and to regulate body processes.

The science of nutrition deals with food values, its digestion, absorption, metabolism in the body and transportation to the tissues for utilisation in growth, development and health promotion in an individual. Nutrition has been established as one of the most important environmental factors affecting health of an individual, the family, the community, the society and the nation.

Functions of Food

Important functions of food include :

(i) It provides energy in the form of heat, for mechanical work etc. Even while the body is at rest some energy is utilized on respiratory, circulatory and other body processes.

(ii) It is essential for the growth of the body and for the repair of daily wear and tear of tissues. Even after the growth is stopped, the body continues to change throughout life and tissues are also changed.

(iii) It is essential for maintenance and regulation of tissue functions, and body temperature.

(iv) It provides the power to the body to build resistance against infections and diseases.

(v) It is essential to satisfy the hunger.

Classification of Food

Man is omnivorous. He selects his food from animal and vegetable origin because the structure and functions of his body are such that it easily digests and metabolises their products. He may be vegetarian or non-vegetarian but his food generally consists of :

(i) Carbohydrates
(ii) Proteins
(iii) Fats
(iv) Mineral salts
(v) Vitamins
(vi) Water

Other Articles of Food Include

(i) Fish

    (ii) Meat

    (iii) Egg

    (iv) Milk

    (v) Condiment and spices

    (vi) Vegetable oils

    (vii) Fruits

    (viii) Vegetables

The above mentioned food articles are used in two ways :

  (a) Substances or products which can be used as such like fruits, dry fruits, radish, carrot, tomato etc.

  (b) Substances or products which can be used by altering their taste by cooking and making them more palatable by adding salt, chillies, spices, vegetable oil etc.

Food may be classified as follows :

1. According to origin :

    (i) From animal sources e.g. meat, fish, egg, milk, butter etc.

    (ii) From vegetable sources e.g. carbohydrates, fruits, dry fruits, vegetables, oils etc.

    (iii) From minerals e.g. mineral salts.

2. According to functions :

    (i) Energy yielding foods such as carbohydrates, fats and oils.

    (ii) Body building foods such as foods rich in proteins like meat, fish, eggs, milk, pulses, oil seeds etc.

    (iii) Protective foods such as foods rich in proteins, vitamins and minerals e.g. milk, green leafy vegetables etc. Protective foods are so called because they protect the body against infections, diseases and ill health.

3. According to nutritive value :

    (i) Animal foods

    (ii) Fats and oils

    (iii) Vegetables

    (iv) Fruits

    (v) Cereals

(vi) Pulses (legumes)

(vii) Nuts and oil seeds

(viii) Sugar

(ix) Condiments and spices

(x) Miscellaneous food articles

4. According to chemical composition

(i) Carbohydrates

(ii) Proteins

(iii) Fats

(iv) Mineral salts

(v) Vitamins

(vi) Water

Classification of food according to chemical composition is more appropriate hence discussed in detail.

(I) CARBOHYDRATES

As the name indicates carbohydrates consist of carbon, hydrogen and oxygen. Carbohydrates are the cheapest and main source of energy as 1 gm of carbohydrates, upon oxidation yields about 4 calories of energy. Poor man's diet consists of 90% carbohydrates, while rich man's diet consists of about 50% carbohydrates. On an average the diet has 55-65% carbohydrates.

Sources of Carbohydrates : The main sources of carbohydrates include wheat, rice, maize, barley, cereals, potatoes, sweet potatoes, turnips, roots and vegetables which are rich in starch while sugar cane, beetroot, honey and fruits are rich in sugars.

Carbohydrates are present in good quantities in food. All carbohydrates have to be changed into glucose and fructose before they are absorbed into the body by means of juices present in the gastrointestinal tract. In the active muscles, the glucose is oxidised for the production of heat and energy. About half of the energy required by the body is met with the carbohydrates. Glucose which cannot be used immediately is converted into glycogen and stored in the liver and muscles or converted into fat which is stored under the skin. The daily requirement of carbohydrates is 400-500 gm.

Functions of Carbohydrates

(a) They are the main source of energy.

(b) They serve as roughage.

(c) They facilitate the bowel evacuation.

Fibres (Roughage)

Fibres mainly consist of cellulose and other complex carbohydrates which are found in fruits, vegetables, legumes, nuts and coarse cereals. It is the indigestible part of food which is partly digested by micro-organisms present in large intestines.

Functions

1. Because it is not digested so passes unchanged through the small intestines and stimulates bowel movements thus acts as mild laxative.

2. It increases the bulk of the diet thus helps to satisfy hunger.

3. It lowers blood cholesterol level thus decreasing the risk of coronary heart diseases.

4. Since it increases the bulk of diet therefore decreases overeating thus helps in preventing obesity.

The daily requirement of fibres is considered to be 20 gm. Shortage of fibres may produce constipation hence plenty of salad should be consumed. They do not have any nutritional value.

(II) PROTEINS

Proteins are the most essential of all the nutrients of food and are necessary for overall growth and repair processes of body tissues. Tissues, muscles, organs, enzymes and hormones are protein in nature. Due to this reason, proteins are of great importance in food. They are composed of carbon, hydrogen, oxygen, nitrogen, phosphorous and sulphur in varying amounts. Proteins differ from carbohydrates and fats that they contain nitrogen.

Proteins are made up of simple compounds known as amino acids. There are 22 known amino acids which are needed by the body. Out of them 10 are such which cannot be synthesised in the body, but are otherwise essential for the body and must be supplied in the food. These are termed as essential amino acids. These essential amino acids are:

1. Leucine
2. Isoleucine
3. Lysine
4. Methionine
5. Phenylalanine
6. Threonine
7. Tryptophane
8. Valine
9. Arginine
10. Histidine

Arginine and histidine are required for growing children. Some authorities do not include these two in the list of essential amino acids. Non-essential amino acids are those which can be synthesized in the body. Examples of such amino acids include alanine, aspartic acid, cystine, glutemic acid, glycine, proline, tyrosine etc.

During the process of digestion the proteins are broken down in gastrointestinal tract by enzymes into simpler amino acids, which are absorbed and pass on to the liver where these amino acids again combine to form the proteins needed by the body.

Sources of Proteins

Proteins are available from two sources i.e. animal and plant sources.

1. Protein rich animal sources include milk, cheese, eggs, meat, fish etc.
2. Protein rich plant sources include pulses, cereals, beans, nuts, grams and soyabeans. These sources contain as much as 25 to 40% protein because of which they are called 'poor man's meat'.

From nutritional point of view, animal proteins are considered superior to vegetable proteins because they contain all the essential amino acids needed by the body but animal proteins are relatively costlier and everybody can't afford it. Moreover, on religious grounds certain communities in India do not take animal proteins. On the other hand vegetable proteins are cheaper and readily available but they are usually deficient in one or more of the essential amino acids needed by the body hence they are considered inferior to animal proteins. A mixed diet containing both animal and vegetable proteins meet the needs of essential amino acids required by the body. Each gm of protein on oxidation yields 4.1 calories of heat, but generally the body depends for its energy on carbohydrates and fats rather than proteins.

Functions of Proteins

Proteins are needed by the body :

(i) For growth and development.

(ii) For repair and maintenance of body tissues.

(iii) For maintenance of osmotic pressure.

(iv) For the synthesis of antibodies, hormones, enzymes, haemoglobin and plasma proteins.

Protein Requirements

The daily requirement of protein for an adult is about 1.0 gm/kg body weight; and it is desirable that one fifth of it should be animal protein. Body requirements of proteins are greater in infancy, pregnancy and lactation when new tissues are formed. The body cannot store excess protein, the body utilizes what it needs and the excess protein is utilized as body fuel. The nitrogenous waste of this protein is excreted by the kidneys.

Effects of Protein Deficiency

The deficiency of proteins in pregnancy may lead to still birth, low birth weight, anaemic baby, mentally retarded and under developed child. In adults it may lead to loss of weight, under weight, anaemia, increased susceptibility to infection, weak muscles, general lethargy, delay in wound healing, oedema and loose stools. Prolonged protein deficiency may cause death of large number of liver cells (i.e. liver necrosis).

(III) FATS

Fats are composed of carbon, hydrogen and oxygen. They differ from carbohydrates that the percentage of these elements is different and there is less of oxygen in fats than in carbohydrates. There are many kinds of fats. Some fats such as groundnut oil and vegetable oil are liquid at room temperature and some fats such as ghee or butter are semisolid or solid in nature. Chemically fats are composed of glycerol and fatty acids. The latter may be saturated or unsaturated. In general animal fats contains saturated fatty acids and glycerin. It is found in eggs, meat, cheese, milk, butter and oily fishes. The vegetable fats contain the unsaturated fatty acids and glycerin. It is found in margarin and vegetable oils.

Fats are also called concentrated sources of heat and energy as 1 gm of fat yields 4 calories of heat on oxidation thus yield more than double the energy as compared to carbohydrates. Human body can synthesize triglycerides and cholesterol endogenously but those fatty acids which cannot be synthesized in the body are known as essential fatty acids which must be incorporated in the diet. Examples include linoleic acid and linolenic acid etc. which are mostly found in vegetable oils.

As fats are insoluble in water, during the process of digestion they are converted into an emulsion for their absorption into the body. Liquid fats and those which melt at body temperature are better digested than those which are much harder. A fat rich diet slows the process of digestion and gives a feeling of heaviness and fullness. In the body, the fat which cannot be immediately used is partly deposited as adipose tissue under the skin and the rest unabsorbed is excreted along with the faeces.

Sources of Fats

(a) Animal sources include ghee, butter, meat, fish oils etc.

(b) Vegetable sources include various vegetable oils such as ground-nut oil, mustard oil, cottonseed oil, sunflower oil, coconut oil etc.

Functions of Fats

The functions of fat are :

1. They are the concentrated source of energy and provide double the energy than that of carbohydrates and proteins. They provide energy especially in starvation.

2. They act as carriers for fat soluble vitamins e.g. vitamins A, D, E & K.

3. They provide support to many organs of the body e.g. heart, kidneys eyes and intestines etc.
4. They supply essential fatty acids which are not found in the body.
5. Fat is used in the formation of cholesterol and steroidal hormones.
6. Fatty layer below the skin play, an important role in maintaining our body temperature thus protects the body from excessive heat and cold.
7. They increase the palatability of food and foods containing fats are tasty.

Effect of Deficiency of Fats

Deficiency of essential fatty acids may lead to rough and dry skin or toad skin. The skin is lustreless and may cause skin lesions.

Excessive intake of animal fats may lead to obesity. It may also lead of increase in blood cholesterol level which may be a contributory factor for the development of heart diseases.

(IV) MINERAL SALTS

The body has about 24 mineral substances which are mainly obtained from food. Many of them are widely distributed in foodstuffs, so a well balanced diet will supply them in sufficient amounts needed by the body. These mineral salts are very essential for the maintenance and growth of the body. They form about 1/20th of body weight.

Minerals are classified into two major groups :
(a) Major minerals e.g. calcium, phosphorus, sodium, potassium etc.
(b) Trace elements e.g. iron, iodine, fluorine, zinc, cobalt etc. These are required in microquantities.

Functions of Mineral Salts

Mineral salts are used to perform the following functions :
1. They constitute and maintain rigid structure of the body such as bones and teeth etc. e.g. calcium, magnesium, phosphorous.

2. They form the part of every cell.

3. They maintain tone and proper function of muscles, nerves and body fluids e.g. calcium and iron.

4. They help in maintaining acid-alkali balance e.g. sodium and potassium chlorides.

5. They stimulate digestive secretions. .

6. They help in general growth of the body.

Some of the most important mineral salts from nutrition point of view are as follows :

1. Calcium

Calcium is very important mineral element of the body. It forms 1.5 to 2% of the body weight, out of which about 99% is found in the bones.

Functions of Calcium

(i) It gives rigidity and strength to the bones.

(ii) It gives hardness and shine to the teeth.

(iii) It controls rythmic activities of heart and contractile muscles.

(iv) It is essential for the clotting of blood.

Sources of Calcium

The best source of calcium is milk. It is also found in cheese, eggs, dark green leafy vegetables, dried beans and fruits. The calcium present in vegetables is not completely absorbed because of the presence of oxalic acid in vegetables which forms an insoluble substance with calcium i.e. calcium oxalate, however calcium present in milk is easily absorbed.

Requirement of Calcium

The daily requirement of calcium for an adult is 0.5 to 1.0 gm. Children, pregnant and lactating mothers need more calcium intake than average adults.

The deficiency of calcium leads to poor development of bones and teeth. It may lead to rickets in children and osteomalacia in adults and delayed blood coagulation.

2. Phosphorus

Phosphorus is contained in every cell of the body. It is essential for the multiplication of cells and overall growth of the body. It is found in cheese, egg yolk, almonds, nuts, peas, beans, whole wheat, liver, milk, spinach, potatoes etc.

The daily requirement of phosphorus is 1.5 gm and increases in pregnancy.

The deficiency of phosphorus leads to softening of bones, caries of teeth and depression of vital processes.

3. Sodium

Sodium chloride is essential for life as it occurs in all tissues and body fluids. It is found in many foods and is also added to food during cooking. It maintains pH, helps in contraction of muscles and in the transmission of nerve impulses in the nerve fibres. Its daily intake varies from 5-20gms.Excess amount of it is excreted through urine and sweat. The deficiency of sodium chloride leads to cramps, marked general weakness, dryness of mouth and mental lassitude. These symptoms can be delayed or even prevented by drinking water containing 0.25% sodium chloride. A high intake of sodium chloride is harmful in congestive heart failure and kidney failure.

4. Potassium

Like sodium, potassium is also very essential for life as it helps in maintaining the pH of various body fluids, helps in contraction of muscles and in the transmission of nerve impulses. It is found in almost every type of food. The daily intake of potassium chloride varies from 5 to 7 gms. The excess is excreted in urine.

5. Iron

Iron is essential for the formation of haemoglobin in red blood cells. It acts as an oxygen carrier to the lungs and tissues and plays an important part in the oxidation and catalysis of enzymes. The total amount of iron present in the body is estimated to be about 3 to 4 gms and 75% of this amount is found in haemoglobin.

The chief sources of iron are liver, red meat, eggs, pulses, cereals, lettuce, dry fruits, dates, figs, milk and dark green leafy vegetables.

Cooking in iron utensils may also contribute significantly in the supply of iron. The daily requirement of iron is 15 mg but an adult woman needs more of iron to compensate for loss of blood in menstruation and also in pregnancy and lactation.

The deficiency of iron leads to anaemia. Anaemic persons are usually more susceptible to the attack of infections. Iron deficiency is a major cause of premature births and large number of neonatal deaths.

6. Iodine

Iodine occurs in all the tissues and fluids of the body. It is an essential constituent of thyroid gland where it is required for the formation of a hormone 'thyroxine' needed for regulating the metabolism.

The chief sources of iodine are seafish, cod liver oil, egg yolk, onions and fresh vegetables. Iodised table salt is used to supply the additional quantity of iodine needed by the body. The daily requirement of iodine for an adult person is 0.15 to 0.30 mg. Its deficiency leads to 'goitre' (swelling of thyroid gland in the neck). Goitre is a common health problem almost throughout India specially in the sub-Himalayan region therefore the government is supplying the 'iodised salt' for eating purposes and the use of common salt for eating purposes is almost banned.

7. Fluorine

Fluorine is an essential element for the dental enamel and for normal mineralisation of bones. The main source of fluorine is drinking water. It is also found in seafish, cheese and tea. Deficiency of fluorine leads to dental caries but on the other hand excessive intake of fluorine leads to formation of patches of brown pigments on the teeth enamel and skeletal fluorosis a crippling disease.

8. Zinc

Zinc is a component of many enzymes. It is required for the synthesis of insulin in pancreas. It is found in meat, fish and milk. Daily requirement is 10-15 mg. which is provided by human diet. Deficiency of zinc leads to retarded growth, delayed healing of wounds, multiple infections and impaired sexual functions.

(V) VITAMINS

Vitamins are complex organic chemical substances which are very essential for normal growth and development of the body. They do not supply energy like fats or carbohydrates but enable the body to use other nutrients. They act as protectives to the body against ill health, infection and disease. They are required in minute quantities and act as catalysts. Generally well balanced diet provides all the necessary vitamins needed by the body but if diet devoid of vitamins is taken for long time it may lead to certain vitamin deficiency diseases which may ultimately lead to death.

Originally these chemical substances were known as 'vitamine' because they were known to be vital for life and were all believed to be amines. But later on it was found that they have diversified structures and some of them do not contain even nitrogen then they were given the name vitamin by Professor J.C. Drummond in the year 1920.

During deficiency of vitamins (avitaminosis) additional quantities of vitamins are required. Avitaminosis usually arises from :

1. Poor intake of vitamins in the diet.
2. Poor absorption from G.I.T. during gastritis, prolonged diarrhoea or drug treatment.
3. Diseases of liver and biliary tract e.g. obstructive jaundice.
4. Chronic alcoholism, malabsorption, allergy and improper digestion due to poor teeth or due to any other reason.

A well balanced diet provides all the vitamins required by the body but the demand of vitamins increases during growth, pregnancy, lactation, prolonged illness and under stress which is met by supplying additional quantities of vitamins to the body.

Classification of Vitamins

Vitamins are classified into two major groups as given below :

1. Fat soluble vitamins e.g. vitamin A, D, E and K.
2. Water soluble vitamins e.g. vitamin B complex and vitamin C. Vitamin B complex includes vitamin B_1, vitamin B_2, vitamin B_6, nicotinic acid, pantothenic acid, folic acid and vitamin B_{12}.

1. FAT SOLUBLE VITAMINS

(a) Vitamin A

It is a fat soluble vitamin and chemically known as 'retinol'. It is essential for maintaining the integrity of the epithelial linings throughout the body for new cell growth and for visual purple. It is anti-infective and growth promoting vitamin. The daily requirement of vitamin A for an adult is 5000 I.U. which increases for growing children and during puberty, pregnancy and lactation from 6000-8000 I.U.

Sources of Vitamin A

Animal sources — Cod liver oil and shark liver oil are the richest sources of vitamin A. It is also available in milk, butter, ghee, eggs and fish.

Vegetable sources — Provitamin A known as carotene is present in abundance in yellow pigment of plants, which is converted into vitamin A in the walls of the intestine. It may be noted that carotenes are the main source of vitamin A for Indians. Vegetable sources of vitamin A include green leafy vegetables, carrots, cabbage, mango and papaya.

Deficiency of Vitamin A

The deficiency of vitamin A leads to :
1. Retarded growth and lowered resistance to bacterial infection.
2. Night blindness (poor adaptation in darkness).
3. Xerophthalmia (dryness of the eye) and keratomalacia of the cornea (black portion of the eye) becomes soft and gets perforated and loses its transparency. This condition is very serious and may result in blindness.
4. Dryness of skin.
5. Respiratory infections like common cold, bronchitis etc.
6. Faulty development of teeth and spongy gums.

Large doses of vitamin A 'Hypervitaminosis A' may lead to loss of weight, dryness of skin, loss of hair, ulceration in the eyes, spontaneous fracture, reduction of ascorbic acid content in the tissues, haemorrhage and lowering of plasma thrombin.

(b) Vitamin D

There are two biological precursors (provitamins) to vitamin D known as ergosterol and 7-dehydro-cholesterol which are converted to vitamin D_2 (ergocalciferol) and vitamin D_3 (cholecalciferol) respectively by ultraviolet rays present in sunlight.

Vitamin D is essential for the calcification of bones and teeth and for the prevention and cure of rickets and osteomalacia. It is thermostable and resistant to oxidation.

Sources of Vitamin D

It is present in egg yolk, cod liver oil, halibut liver oil, butter and ghee. Cod liver oil is the richest source of vitamin D. Sunlight is an important natural source of vitamin D. The ultraviolet rays present in sunlight convert ergosterol found in skin to vitamin D_2 and vitamin D_3. The rate at which vitamin D is synthesised in the skin depends upon the exposure of the body to the sun.

The daily requirement of vitamin D is 1000 I.U.

Deficiency of Vitamin D

Deficiency of vitamin D leads to rickets and dental caries in children and osteomalacia in adults. It may also lead to increased loss of calcium and phosphates in the faeces.

Excess amount of vitamin D leads to hypercalcaemia resulting in anorexia (loss of appetite), nausea, vomiting, drowziness and even coma.

(c) Vitamin E

Vitamin E (tocopherol) is an anti-sterility vitamin. It was discovered by Dr. Evans of U.S.A. who named it vitamin E. It is a fat soluble vitamin which is stable to heat and light but is destroyed on oxidation.

Sources

Vitamin E is present in wheat, cereal embryos, green leaves and some vegetable oils. Vitamin E is widely distributed in nature therefore its deficiency is rarely noticed.

Therapeutically vitamin E is used in the prevention of abortion, in certain menstrual disorders and in the improvement of lactation. It plays an important role in the maintenance of structural and functional features of smooth muscles, cardiac muscles and skeletal muscles.

Deficiency of vitamin E leads to death of foetus in uterus and sterility in males and females in the lower animals. The daily requirement of vitamin E for an adult is 10 mg.

(d) Vitamin K

Vitamin K is a fat soluble vitamin. It is stable to heat. It is essential for normal coagulation of blood and necessary for the formation of pro-thrombin and other blood clotting factors in the liver. Vitamin K occurs in two forms i.e. vitamin K_1 and K_2. Vitamin K_1 is naturally available in alfalfa plant and vitamin K_2 is isolated from putrefied fish meal and is also synthesized by the intestinal bacteria.

Sources

It occurs in green leaves, alfalfa, spinach, cauliflower, cabbage, carrot - tops etc. Bacteria present in the intestine also produces required amount of vitamin K. Administration of antibiotics for more than a week may cause deficiency of vitamin K due to supression of bacteria present in the intestines.

Deficiency of vitamin K leads to increased prothrombin time (hypoprothrombinemia) and a tendency for haemorrhage from skin due to prolongation of blood clotting.

2. WATER SOLUBLE VITAMINS

The vitamins included in this group are water soluble which include B-complex and vitamin C. The vitamin B was classified as vitamin B-complex because they tend to occur together in foods in relatively high concentrations. Since the identity of each vitamin had been established so the term B-complex is no longer appropriate. The vitamin B group includes vitamin B_1, B_2, B_6 nicotinic acid, pantothenic acid, folic acid and vitamin B_{12}.

(a) Vitamin B₁

Vitamin B_1 is also known as thiamine and aneurine hydrochloride. It is soluble in water and alcohol but insoluble in fat solvents. It is relatively stable to heat but is destroyed in neutral or alkaline solution.

It is essential for the normal growth and health of the body and also plays an important part in carbohydrate metabolism.

Sources

Thiamine is widely distributed in small amounts in all natural foods. The main sources are rice polishing, unmilled cereals, pulses, nuts, yeast, egg yolk, fish, meat etc. It has been synthesised and has been obtained in crystalline form from rice polishings and wheat embryos.

Thiamine is readily lost during milling of rice, wheat and cereals and also during the process of washing and cooking of pulses.

Deficiency

Deficiency of vitamin B_1 leads to beri beri, neuritis, loss of appetite, atony (muscles lacking their normal elasticity) of G.I.T; mental depression, anaemia, enlarged heart and increased palpitation on slight exertion etc.

The daily requirement of vitamin B_1 is 2 mg which increases in shock, haemorrhage, regular haemodialysis and serious illness. The body content of thianine is 30 mg and if more than this is given it is merely lost in urine.

(b) Vitamin B_2

Vitamin B_2 is also known as riboflavin. It is a water soluble yellow pigment closely related to flavins. It is concerned with normal protein, carbohydrate and fat metabolism. It is associated as coenzyme in tissue oxidation and respiration.

Sources

Vitamin B_2 is found in yeast, milk, eggs, liver, kidney and green vegetables. Wheat, millets and pulses also contain good amount but rice is a poor source of vitamin B_2. Germinating pulses also provide this vitamin. Vitamin B_2 is synthesised by bacteria in the large intestine which is an additional source.

Deficiency

The deficiency of riboflavin leads to angular stomatitis, glossitis (soreness of the tongue), redress and burning sensation in the eyes, dermatitis, poor wound healing process, photophobia and retardation of growth.

The daily requirement of riboflavin is 2-3 mg.

(c) Niacin

(Nicotinic acid, nicotinamide, vitamin B_3 or vitamin P.P. i.e. pellagra preventing factor).

The term niacin is collectively used to represent both nicotinic acid (niacin) and nicotinamide (Niacinamide) which posseses pellagra preventing (P.P.) factor. It acts as co-enzyme for fat, protein and carbohydrate metabolism and for tissue respiration.

Sources

Foods rich in niacin are whole grain cereals, pulses, nuts, meat, liver, yeast and green vegetables.

Deficiency

Deficiency of niacin leads to pellagra known as three D's disease which represents diarrhoea, dermatitis and dementia (related to brain disease). In severe deficiency it may lead to pigmentation of the skin specially in the regions of the skin exposed to sunlight like hands, feet, face and neck. It also leads to ·weakness, anorexia, insomnia and mental depression. Pellagra is found in those areas where maize and jowar is the main source of food.

The daily requirement of niacin is about 12-18 mg. In deficiency diseases it may be given upto 50 mg daily.

(d) Vitamin B₆

Vitamin B_6 is also known as pyridoxine. It exists in three forms i.e. pyridoxine, pyridoxal and pyridoxamine. The term pyridoxine is collectively used to represent all the three forms which are interconvertible and have the same biological activity. It is essential for metabolism of amino acids, fats and carbohydrates. It is necessary for haemoglobin synthesis and also as an anti dermatitis factor.

Sources

It is present in liver, egg yolk, fish, whole cereals, yeast, wheat germs and leafy vegetables.

Deficiency

The deficiency of vitamin B_6 is rarely observed in human beings because enough pyridoxine is present in diet consumed by man. Deficiency leads to epileptiform convulsions. This may be due to lack of Gamma aminobutyric acid (GABA) whose formation is dependent on vitamin B_6. Its deficiency may also lead to dermatitis, glossitis and skin lesions.

The daily requirement of pyridoxine is about 2 mg.

(e) Folic Acid (Vitamin M)

Folic acid is also known as vitamin M and folacin. It is essential for the synthesis of DNA (deoxyribo nucleic acid) in the nuclei of the cells. It stimulates blood formation and take part in maturation of red blood cells. It is extensively used in macrocytic and pernicious anaemia.

Sources

Folic acid is present in liver, kidneys, yeast and green leafy vegetables.

Deficiency

Deficiency of folic acid leads to disturbances in the synthesis of DNA. It also leads to megaloblastic anaemia, gastrointestinal disturbances like diarrhoea, distention and flatulence. Anaemia usually occurs during pregnancy as nutritional deficiency anaemia.

The daily requirement of folic acid is 100-300 μg.

(f) Vitamin B_{12}

Vitamin B_{12} is also known as cyanocobalamin and is an antipernicious anaemia factor. Due to the presence of cobalt it is red crystalline or amorphous powder soluble in water.

Vitamin B_{12} is essential for the normal functioning of all cells but particularly for cells of the bone marrow, the nervous system and the G.I.T. It is also necessary for the synthesis of DNA. It plays an important part in the carbohydrate, fat and protein metabolism. It is essential for the formation and maturation of red blood cells.

Sources

Vitamin B_{12} is found in animal sources like liver, eggs, fish, beef and milk. Foods of vegetable origin do not contain this vitamin. Therefore deficiency of vitamin B_{12} is noticed in those patients who are strict vegetarians. Vitamin B_{12} is isolated from aqueous liver extracts and from *Streptomyces griseus.* Commercially it is obtained from the fermentation of the latter source.

Deficiency

Deficiency of vitamin B_{12} leads to pernicious anaemia (anaemia due to marked decrease in number of RBCs) and lack of intrinsic factor. It also affects the nervous system including the spinal cord. The deficiency of vitamin B_{12} is to some extent linked with the deficiency of another vitamin i.e. folic acid.

The initial dose of vitamin B_{12} is 30 μg to 1 mg by intramuscular injection which should be repeated at suitable intervals of time. In pernicious anaemia vitamin B_{12} when given orally is not absorbed in effective amounts unless it is accompanied by intrinsic factors hence must be administered parenterally in micro quantities.

It is a very costly vitamin since about a ton of liver is required to prepare only 20-25 mg of vitamin B_{12}.

(g) Biotin

It is also known as vitamin B_7 or vitamin H. It acts as a co-enzyme for the metabolism of fat and carbohydrates. It is found in liver, eggs, yeast, cereals and vegetables.

In human beings the deficiency of biotin rarely occurs but if deficiency occurs it leads to dermatitis, eczema, muscle ache, lethargy, anorexia and nausea.

Daily requirement of biotin is 100-300 μg.

(h) Choline

It cannot be considered as true vitamin because it does not function as a co-enzyme in any of the biochemical reactions. Moreover unlike vitamins it is required in quite large amounts to exert its effects. From various metabolic studies it has been found out that choline is important, if not essential for the infant. Therefore it is necessary that choline must be present in infant formulas at least to the level found in human milk.

Sources

Foods which contain large amount of choline are liver, kidney, meat, fish, nuts, beans, peas and eggs. Moderate amount is present in cereals, milk, and a number of vegetables.

Deficiency

Deficiency of choline causes deposition of fat in liver, degeneration of liver and kidneys.

An average mixed diet is estimated to contain 500 to 900 mg choline per day which is considered adequate for human beings.

The other vitamins of B group include inositol and para-amino benzoic acid (PABA). The deficiency of these two vitamins rarely occurs because normal diet contains sufficient amount of inositol and PABA.

(i) Vitamin C

Vitamin C is also known as ascorbic acid and anti-scorbutic vitamin. It is water soluble. Ascorbic acid is the most unstable of all the vitamins being readily destroyed by exposure to air and heat. It is also destroyed on preservation of fruits.

Functions

1. It is essential for the maintenance of cellular structure and for the synthesis of collagen, the protein substance that binds the cells together; if collagen is not formed, healing of wounds will be delayed.
2. It is essential for the maturation of red blood corpuscles.
3. It plays an important role in tissue oxidation.
4. It helps in checking the bleeding phenomenon.
5. It increases the absorption of iron.
6. It increases the general resistance of the body to fight infections.
7. It is involved in the synthesis of adrenal hormones.

Sources of Vitamin C

The main sources of vitamin C are fresh fruits and vegetables like orange, lemon, tomato, papaya, potato, cabbage, cauliflower, spinach, bean, pulses and germinating cereals. Amla and guava are very rich sources of vitamin C. The fresh juice of Amla contains nearly twenty times as much vitamin C as orange juice and a single fruit of Amla is equivalent in vitamin content to one to two oranges. Vitamin C has been isolated in pure form from fruit juice and has also been synthetically manufactured. Animal foods like milk, meat, fish etc. are poor sources of vitamin C.

Deficiency of Vitamin C

Deficiency of vitamin C leads to scurvy, anaemia, dental caries, offensive breath, spongy gums, loss of weight, delayed wound healing and tendency to haemorrhage. The bones become brittle and cease to grow. If bone fracture occurs it heals very slowly. In vitamin C deficiency there is increased susceptibility to infections.

Scurvy is characterised by :

1. Weakness and fatigue with muscular and joint pain, breathlessness and tachycardia.
2. The gums become spongy, inflammed and bleed easily. The teeth get loosened from sockets.
3. There is frequent haemorrhages and patient is anaemic.
4. There is increased susceptibility to infection.
5. In severe cases of scurvy previous wounds may break down and become open wounds again.
6. Prolonged deficiency of vitamin C may ultimately lead to death.

The daily requirement of vitamin C is 30-60 mg which increases in disease, pregnancy, and lactation. For therapeutic use it is given 200-500 mg per day orally. For treating scurvy it is given 1-2 gm per day. Since vitamin C cannot be stored in the body so a daily intake of recommended dose is necessary for good health.

(VI) WATER

Water is the most important constituent of food for all living bodies. A man can live without food for a number of days but in the absence of water it is impossible for him to survive beyond a few days. Human body contains about 70% of water. All tissues, organs and bones contain water.

Water is present in all types of foods like vegetables, fruits, milk etc. in varying proportions. But the water available from these sources is not sufficient to meet the body requirements, therefore water must be taken either plain or in the form of various drinks like tea, coffee, milk, juice, squash and other beverages. A small amount of water is also formed in the tissues as a result of metabolism.

Functions of Water

1. Water is an essential constituent of body fluids like blood, lymph, cerebrospinal fluid (CSF) etc.
2. It helps in the regulation of body temperature by evaporation through skin and lungs.
3. It serves as a vehicle for solution and dilution of solid foods, whereby these are easily digested and metabolised.
4. It is essential to make up the loss caused by its excretion in urine, sweat, breath, milk in lactating mothers and to some extent in faeces.
5. It helps in the transport of nutrients within the body.
6. It helps in excreting the waste products from the body.
7. It is important in building and repair of body tissues.

Requirement of Water

The water requirement varies from person to person, atmospheric temperature and the manual labour done by the individual. With rise in atmospheric temperature and humidity of air the necessity of water intake increases. People living in hot countries like India need more water than people living in cold countries. The requirement of water is more in manual labourers. The water intake and water loss must be equal in order to maintain the normal water balance. Inadequate intake of water creates circulatory disturbances, disturbance in heat regulation mechanism, retention of metabolic products and less secretion of urine. On the other hand abundant intake of water promotes the circulation of fluids and increases the activity of kidneys with free secretion of urine.

Excessive water loss from the body as in the case of severe diarrhoea and vomitting leads to dehydration and water retention as in the case of kidney failure leads to oedema.

On an average a normal healthy person daily needs 6 glasses of water for drinking and it is estimated that about 2.27 litres of water enters the body as such or in the form of food or cold drinks etc. out of which about 1.37-1.81 litres is excreted in urine, sweat, faeces etc. Therefore to keep the body healthy plenty of water must be taken daily.

Balanced Diet

The food taken by human beings is called diet. A diet which contains adequate amounts of all the essential nutrients like carbohydrates, proteins, fats, minerals and vitamins sufficient for the normal growth and development of the body, is called a balanced diet. A balanced diet should also contain sufficient amounts of water and roughage material. In addition, the food should satisfy the taste and desire of a person.

No single food can provide us all the essential nutrients needed by our body in adequate amounts. So, we have to choose a number of food items which are taken together to provide all nutrients, water and roughage to the body. The various constituents of balanced diet perform different functions as described below :

1. Carbohydrates and fats provide energy to the body.
2. Proteins provide material for growth and development of the body, and repair of damaged tissues.
3. Mineral salts help the body to form blood, bones, teeth and to regulate body functions.
4. Vitamins are needed in the diet to catalyse certain chemical reactions in the body which are necessary for normal growth and maintenance of good health.
5. Water is essential in the diet to carry out various life processes in the body like digestion, metabolism, transport, excretion and regulation of body temperature.
6. Roughage is required in the diet for proper digestion, proper peristaltic movements and bowel evacuation.

The composition of a balanced diet for an average adult male is given below :

Cereals (Atta, rice)	400 gm.
Pulses	50-85 gm.
Oil or ghee	57 gm.
Leafy vegetables	114 gm.

Other vegetables	85 gm.
Root vegetables	85 gm.
Fruits	85 gm.
Milk and milk products	284 gm.
Sugar and jaggery	57 gm.
Fish/meat	85 gm.
Eggs	1-2 eggs
Water	according to need
Salt and condiments	according to taste

There is no universal rule for balanced diet. It can be changed according to one's taste, culture, local and seasonal availability of diet articles and climatic conditions of the place. But as far as possible the basic nutrient ingredients must be present in balanced diet.

Unbalanced Diet

Since India is a poor country, majority of the population live below the poverty line and they don't get proper food to eat. Generally a large population depends on unbalanced diet having the following deficiencies:

1. Mostly the diet is composed of carbohydrates (about 90%) and contains very less amount of proteins especially derived from animal origin.
2. There is less amount of fats, especially animal fat.
3. There is inadequate supply of inorganic materials.
4. There is lack of vitamin A, D and B complex.
5. There is lack of variety and ignorance in proper cooking.

Deficiency of food factors in the diet is the major cause of many diseases like xerophthalmia, beri-beri, rickets, scurvy, endemic goitre, pallegra etc.

From the above deficiencies in diet it is clear that ignorance about balanced diet is the main problem rather than the shortage of food. The people suffer from malnutrition due to protein, iron and vitamin deficiencies in diet which can be easily overcome by making best use of locally available food stuffs and thus help the people suffering from malnutrition. The groundnut, soyabean or black gram flour are quite rich in proteins which can be mixed in 1 : 4 ratio with wheat flour forming what is called fortified flour. The government is supplying such flour rich in protein and vitamins at low cost to the poor people. To meet vitamin and iron deficiencies the use of locally grown leafy vegetables should be encouraged. The agencies like WHO, UNICEF and FAO (Food and Agriculture Organisation) are mainly working to eradicate malnutrition among poor people. Mid-day meals are given to school children free of cost. Vitamins and haematins are supplied free of cost to the needy persons by the government and above mentioned agencies.

Diet for Infants and Children

The dietary needs of an infant below the age of 6 months are met from mother's milk if the mother's milk is adequate. About 600 ml of breast milk is secreted daily by nursing mothers during first 6 months of lactation. This amount of milk is quite sufficient to meet the needs of an infant. The mother's milk is full of nutritional values and contains sufficient antibodies to provide immunity to child from various diseases. Mother's milk is the best food for infants because it provides all the nutrients required by the infants. As it is free from harmful bacteria so chances of gastro-intestinal disturbances are less frequent in breast-fed babies. Mother's milk is easily digested.

After about six months the secretion of breast milk decreases whereas the nutritional requirements of the child increases. Therefore "supplementary feeding" of the infant must be started from the age of 4 months. Such feeding should be rich in protein and other nutrients. These feedings are usually cow's milk, fruit juice, soft cooked rice and vegetables. At the age of one year the child should be given solid foods consisting of cereals, pulses, vegetables and fruits.

It is suggested that breast feeding should be continued as far as possible specially throughout the first year so that the infant continues to get valuable nutrients, proteins and antibodies from mother's milk. Now a days a great stress is laid on breast feeding the infants. In many poor families young children are breast fed until they are 2-3 years old and are not given other foods eaten by the rest of the family which is a wrong practice and results in malnutrition thereby leading to many kinds of diseases.

The growing children from 1 to 5 years of age and school going children show a good deal of physical activity and growth, so they need extra proteins, vitamins and minerals. Therefore diet rich in proteins, vitamins and minerals should be given to growing children. Besides these iron, calcium and phosphorus should be supplied for the formation of blood, for development of bones and better teeth respectively.

Diet for Pregnant and Lactating Mothers

A pregnant woman requires special consideration regarding her diet because she is to feed the two i.e. herself and the embryo. The exact need depends on her general health, stage of pregnancy, weight and daily activities. In addition to balanced diet she should take adequate amount of proteins, carbohydrates, minerals especially iron, calcium, phosphorus and iodine which are needed to perform various functions such as formation of blood and bones for the developing baby in the womb of the mother. She also needs extra dose of vitamins for the baby. A high intake of proteins is essential during second half of pregnancy which will be helpful for the proper development of the baby and also help in promoting the lactation. Low intake of proteins may lead to abortion in pregnant women.

Lactating or nursing mothers (who breast feed their babies) also need a special diet to take care of their additional requirements for feeding the baby. The baby gets its proteins and other essential nutrients from mother's milk. She needs a diet rich of proteins, calcium and vitamins. The proteins should be from animal origin in the form of milk, eggs, fish and meat. But special stress should be laid on milk. Infants require higher amount of vitamin A and B complex so mother's diet should contain higher amount of these vitamins for supply to the infant in breast milk. Breast milk is usually deficient in vitamin C and D which should be given to the infants in the form of cod liver oil and orange juice. A nursing mother should take lot of milk. This will provide sufficient proteins, calcium and vitamins to the baby who will grow and develop as a healthy baby.

Nutritional Deficiency Diseases

The diseases which occur due to deficiencies in nutrition are as under :

Nutrient Deficiency	Diseases
1. Protein deficiency which is also known as protein calorie malnutrition (PCM) or protein energy malnutrition (PEM)	Kwashiorkor and marasmus. Kwashiorkor results due to very low consumption of proteins in the diet. This condition is seen in the case of children of 1-4 years of age. During this condition there is oedema, anaemia retarded growth, loss of appetite, diarrhoea and less hair growth. Marasmus results due to deficiency of proteins, carbohydrates and fats in the diet of infants especially the infants who are deprived of breast milk and fed with diluted cow's milk which is inadequate for normal growth and development of the child. It usually occurs in the age group of 1/2 to 5 years of age. During this condition there is rapid loss of body weight, wasting of muscles, skin becomes loose and ribs of the child look very prominent. These two diseases are the major causes of ill health in poor families throughout the world and death of children occurs before the age of five years. Protein deficiency in adults is also very common in poor families. In adults protein deficiency will result in reduced weight, loose skin, anaemia, greater susceptibility to infection, general lethargy, delay in healing of wounds, oedema and frequent loose motion.
2. Vitamin A	Xerophthalmia, night blindness and keratomalacia.
3. Vitamin D	Rickets and osteomalacia.
4. Vitamin E	Sterility.
5. Vitamin K	Hypoprothrombinaemia (deficiency of clotting factor, prothrombin in the blood resulting in delayed clotting of blood) which further leads to haemorrhages.
6. Vitamin B_1 (Thiamine)	Beri-beri.
7. Vitamin B_2 (Riboflavin)	Angular stomatitis (cracking of the skin at the corners of the mouth), soreness and inflammation of the mouth and tongue.

(Contd.)

Nutrient Deficiency	Diseases
8. P-P factor (Nicotinic acid)	Pellagra with diarrhoea, dermatitis, insomnia and mental depression
9. Vitamin B_6 (Pyridoxine)	Muscular dystrophy, rigidity and dermatitis in rats. In man deficiency of vitamin B_6 is rare.
10. Vitamin B_{12}	Pernicious anaemia (defective produc-tion of red blood cells).
11. Vitamin C (Ascorbic acid)	Scurvy, anaemia, bad teeth, offensive breath, spongy gums, loss of weight, delayed healing of wounds and hae-morrhages.
12. Calcium	Poor development of bones and teeth, rickets, osteomalacia and delayed blood coagulation.
13. Phosphorus	Softening of bones, dental caries, stunted growth and depression of vital organs.
14. Iron	Anaemia
15. Iodine	Goitre
16. Sodium chloride	Cramps, marked general weakness, mental lassitude (uninterested to do work) and feel exhausted.

Problems of over nutrition

1. Over eating	Obesity
2. Excess vitamin A	Hypervitaminosis A causing headache, nausea, vomiting, irritability and anorexia (loss of appetite).
3. Excess vitamin D	Hypervitaminosis D causing anorexia, nausea, vomiting, thirst, polyuria (excessive secretion of urine) and drowsiness. Calcium and phosphorus levels in serum and urine are raised. Calcium may be deposited in many tissues.
4. Sodium chloride	Hypertension and many other cardiac disorders.
5. Fluorine	Discolouring of teeth enamel (called mottling of teeth) and abnormal calcification of bones (deposition of calcium on the bones and teeth which is known as fluorosis).

3

DEMOGRAPHY AND FAMILY PLANNING

DEMOGRAPHY

Demography may be defined as the science which deals with the study of all aspects of population progress, welfare, death in a family, birth in a family, age and number of children, number of school going children, their educational qualifications; sickness, deformities in the family and sanitation etc. It also includes the study of standard of living as well as property held.

The other terms used in place of demography include 'population dynamics' and 'population studies'.

The main sources of demographic data include vital registration system of births and deaths and census. From these demographic studies many statistical conclusions can be drawn as given below :

1. Population of the country in any particular year.
2. Birth rate.
3. Death rate.
4. The difference between birth rate and death rate results in addition to the net population every year.
5. Men-women ratio, married and unmarried.
6. Per capita income.
7. Per capita agriculture land.

8. Nourishment and undernourishment data.
9. Literacy rate.
10. Density of population per sq. km.
11. The distribution of urban and rural population.
12. Religious composition.
13. Life expectation data.

DEMOGRAPHIC CYCLE

From census studies it is found out that about 80% of the world's population is living in the developing countries and the remaining 20% of the world's population is living in developed countries. According to history of population the population growth takes place according to a cycle known as demographic cycle. This cycle is divided into following stages :

(a) **High Stationary Stage :** It is the first stage during which the population remains stationary because there is a high birth rate as well as high death rate which cancel each other hence the population remains stationary.

(b) **Early Expanding Stage :** It is the second stage during which the death rate begins to fall but the birth rate remains unchanged so there is increase in the population. Most of the developing countries like India fall in this stage.

(c) **Late Expanding Stage :** It is the third stage during which the birth rate decreases but still the population continues to increase because the birth rate is still higher than the death rate.

(d) **Low Stationary Stage :** It is the fourth stage during which the population remains almost stationary because there is low birth rate as well as low death rate. Developed countries like America fall in this stage.

(e) **Declining Stage :** It is the fifth stage during which the population begins to decrease because the birth rate is lower than the death rate.

Fertility

The ability to produce child is known as fertility. During this process male and female partner play an equal and active role. The reproductive period in women is roughly from 15-45 years.

In order to control population growth the fertility rate will have to be checked by adopting some suitable methods of family planning.

In certain countries where population is decreasing (declining stage) there fertility-promoting programmes are encouraged rather than fertility control programmes.

Factors on which Fertility Depends

Fertility depends on the following factors :

1. Age of marriage
2. Duration of married life
3. Spacing of children
4. Education
5. Economic stutus
6. Caste and religion
7. Nutrition
8. Adoption of family planning measures

Population Explosion in India

The population of our country is increasing at an alarming rate and according to population studies India has become the second largest country in the world, accounting for 15% of the world's population with only 2.4% of the world's land area. In the beginning of 20th century the population of India was 23.8 crores but in the year 1994 it was about 90 crores. The Indian population is increasing by about 25 millions every year. It means more than 70,000 babies are born every day.

If population growth rate goes on increasing and remains unchecked then it may cross 1000 million mark by the end of 2000 A.D. and will become the world's first country in population as compared to China. This population explosion is needed to be controlled in order to avoid its adverse effects on the country's economical, social and environmental aspects.

Previously the growth of population was limited because there used to be high death rate due to epidemics, famines (scarcities) and other natural calamities like floods, earthquakes and to some extent wars. But now-a-days the death rate has sharply decreased due to improvement in health services in the fields of maternity and child health (MCH), school health services and control of most of the communicable diseases. With the advancement of technology even some control has been made on natural calamities. Through all these measures though death rate has decreased but birth rate has not appreciably decreased. Thus, it will be seen that it is the high birth rate as compared to low death rate, which is the main cause of population explosion in India.

In under-developed and developing countries the cost of living is increasing day by day. For an average person it has become extremely difficult to meet both ends and one remains always busy in earning his bread and butter. Neither he has spare money nor time to join clubs or other recreational facilities. He remains more attached to his family. For his recreation he indulges in sexual intercourse (for which no money is required) resulting into repeated conceptions and ultimately become helpless when his family grows into a large family. This leads to poverty and unemployment which results into immoral acts and encourage thefts, day robberies and even murders. When a young man or woman will remain unemployed and empty pocket he or she will indulge in such immoral acts. This state of affair is seen in a large section of young people.

Causes of High Birth Rate

1. Early attainment of puberty in girls generally upto 14 years of age.
2. Early marriage even at the age of 15 or below.
3. Poverty and low standard of living.
4. Illiteracy.
5. Lack of recreational facilities due to poverty.
6. Lack of awareness regarding methods of family planning.
7. Due to tradition, superstition and faith that the children are the gift of God and is not the result of man's deeds. This ideology and fate among depressed class in villages is responsible for a large family in poorman's house.

CONSEQUENCES OF POPULATION GROWTH

Population growth has created lot of problems for the public as well as for the government. Some of the serious problems include :

1. Food Problem

Daily a large number of new mouths are added to our existing population which require food for their existence. Though the government has taken a number of measures for increasing the food production which has led to bumper crops in the past few years but even then India has to import food grains.

2. Falling Economic Standards

In spite of allround development in our country the entire economy is being eaten up by rapid growth of population. In India about 40 percent of total population is below 15 years of age or 'young population' whereas about 13 per cent is above 60 years of age. In other words about 55 percent of our population is dependent on the remaining 45 percent for all kinds of their requirements. Therefore dependency burden is very high. Per capita income is very low and more than 40 percent of India's population lives below poverty line. The benefits of planned development are mostly consumed by new population, making it more and more difficult to raise the existing standard of living.

3. Social Problems

The population explosion has led to various social problems which include :

(a) Poverty
(b) Unemployment
(c) Illiteracy due to inadequate schooling facilities
(d) Psychological disturbances due to lack of individual attention towards children in large families
(e) Inadequate or substandard housing facilities
(f) Overcrowding at all places
(g) Law and order problem

4. Health Problems

(a) Repeated pregnancies will deteriorate the health of the mother which may increase maternal mortality rate
(b) Higher infant and child deaths
(c) Lower expectation of life

    (d) Inadequate nutrition

    (e) Poor sanitation and pollution of water, food, soil and air

    (f) Poor health care services. More hospitals, more doctors, more nurses and more financial resources are needed.

5. Ecological Problems

With population explosion we need more land for housing, hospitals, schools and industries etc. For this purpose we will have to destroy the forests which will lead to ecological disturbances in turn leading to natural calamities.

From the above facts it is quite clear that food, social, economic and health problems of the country cannot be successfully tackled till the population growth is controlled.

CONTROL OF OVER POPULATION

The problem of over population can be tackled only if all its aspects are taken into account and public give full co-operation to the government in solving this major problem. Merely advising the couples about the contraceptive methods is not going to help. Keeping this in view the government has started many programmes like maternity and child health services, family planning services. The family planning programme has been converted into family welfare programme with the idea to bring down the infant mortality rate and to improve the maternity services so that there is demand for less children. Family planning services are provided to the eligible couples and follow up of such cases is done carefully to remove all complications, fear and suspicions about family planning.

Though the above mentioned factors will help in checking the population problem but the following measures will also be helpful to a great extent.

1. Raising the Minimum Age of Marriage

If the minimum age of marriage is raised from 15-16 years to 19-20 years there can be reduction in birth rate. Recently the government has raised the minimum age of marriage as 21 years for boys and 18 years for girls. But it should be raised further.

2. Education

If the public is educated they can understand such problems in the proper perspective. For this purpose government and social organisations and students can play a great role.

3. Female Literacy and Increasing Employment Opportunities for Women

If the female are educated they will get better opportunities for employment. Thus with more earning their standard of living will improve and social contacts will widen. The socio-economic status has direct bearing on awareness and practice of family planning.

4. Recreational Facilities

If the recreational facilities are provided at cheaper rates for the poor class, it will also affect the population growth.

5. Decrease in Birth Rate

This is the only possible solution of checking the population explosion and government is laying much stress on family planning methods. Studies have shown that when all births are postponed by one year in each group, there was a decline in total population.

Government alone cannot solve this population problem. All social, religious and charitable organisations, men, women, college students and public in general will have to take part in tackling the population explosion and making the public aware about the advantages of small family norms which can be attained by adopting suitable contraceptive methods.

FAMILY PLANNING

Family planning means to plan and limit the size of the family in accordance with the social, economic and health conditions so as to ensure that the family is happy both physically and mentally.

The term 'family planning' is replaced with a broader term 'family welfare' which is basically related to quality of life. It includes nutrition, health, education, employment, welfare of the women, shelter, safe drinking water etc.

An individual family consists of husband, wife and their children. All the members of a family are dependent on each other for allround health, welfare, physical, mental, social and economical well being. A family constitutes a unit of community and the welfare of a family affects the community, the nation and the humanity at large. Therefore, if the families are small, they will tend to be economically better off and happy which will ultimately affect the nation as a whole.

Most parents in India have very limited economical and social resources for limited number of children in order to give them healthy surroundings.

From puberty to menopause in females and in adult life of a male there is great loss of reproductive cells without sexual union, with sexual union and even after fertilization. If conceptions are too frequent and incompatible with health and economic resources of parents there will be abortions, miscarriages and still births. Even if the child is born he will not get enough care, will be under nourished and in a low state of health. Many of them will die young and others may live handicapped life. Their standard of living and education will also be low and large family will affect health and happiness of each member of the family. Therefore the size of the family should be reduced by adopting any suitable method of family planning.

Factors to be taken into consideration for selection of couples for contraceptive methods :

1. Age of the couple
2. Health of the couple
3. Number of pregnancies the women already had
4. Number of living children
5. Health of the children
6. Sex of the children
7. Age of the youngest child
8. Whether the couple wants to space their children or to limit the size of the family
9. Preference of the couple for a particular method
10. Facilities available in the home e.g. water supply, privacy and regarding storage of contraceptives
11. Cost involved in purchasing contraceptives i.e. free supply or cost to be borne by the user

12. Co-operation and responsibility of either partner
13. Medical advice for using contraceptive method and in certain cases any particular method

Methods of Family Planning or Methods of Birth Control

It is the general tendency that a man wants sexual pleasure and no birth of the child but the woman wants to bear the first child at the earliest and one or two more afterwards. She gets gradually motivated and becomes a fit case for family planning. Still some of the couples in first year of the marriage do not want to produce the child because of sexual pleasure. Child should be produced by choice not by chance. Couples vary in their family planning needs and preferences. Therefore, it is important for family planning programmes to offer as many different methods of fertility regulation as possible so that the people can choose the method most suitable to their needs. Now-a-days a large number of methods of birth control are available out of which the couples may select any method most suitable to their needs and circumstances. These methods include :

A. Temporary methods.
B. Permanent methods.

A. Temporary Methods

1. *Natural methods :*
   (a) Sexual abstinence method
   (b) Coitus interruptus (withdrawal method)
   (c) Safe period (rhythm method)
   (d) Basal body temperature method
   (e) Cervical mucus method
   (f) Prolonged lactation method
   (g) Vaginal washing method

2. *Spacing methods :*
   (i) Barrier contraceptives (mechanical methods)
       (a) Condom
       (b) Diaphragm
       (c) Intrauterine devices
   (ii) Chemical methods
       (a) Foam tablets.

  (b) Contraceptive creams and jellies.
  (c) Soluble tablets (pessaries).
  (d) Oral contraceptives (oral pills)

B. Permanent Methods

  (a) Vasectomy
  (b) Tubectomy
  (c) Laparoscopy
  (d) Medical termination of pregnancy

Table 3.1. Showing contraceptive methods for male and female

S. No.	Male	S. No.	Female
1.	Sexual abstinence method	1.	Sexual abstinence method
2.	Coitus interruptus (withdrawal method)	2.	Safe period (Rhythm method)
		3.	Basal body temperature method
3.	Use of condom	4.	Cervical mucus method
4.	Vasectomy	5.	Prolonged lactation method
		6.	Vaginal washing method
		7.	Diaphragms
		8.	I.U.D.
		9.	Foam tablets
		10.	Contraceptive jellies and creams
		11.	Oral pills
		12.	Tubectomy
		13.	Laparoscopy

A. TEMPORARY METHODS

These methods are used for keeping a space in the birth of the children. That is why these methods are known as spacing methods. These methods can be discontinued easily at any time by the user when a pregnancy is desired. There are different methods for men and women. Some of the temporary methods of birth control are as follows :

1. Natural Methods

Natural methods of contraception are used when the couple is not willing to use any other artificial method either due to medical reasons or due to religious or personal beliefs. These natural methods are very effective methods of family planning if the couples understand how to use natural family planning methods and do not have intercourse during the fertile phase of the menstrual cycle. But if care is not taken during the fertile phase and the couple indulges in intercourse then there are chances for pregnancy to occur.

The natural methods of contraception include :

(a) Sexual Abstinence

Sexual abstinence literally means complete stoppage of sexual contacts. Though it is completely effective method of birth control but it is not practicable at all for married couples and is not considered as a method of contraception applicable to masses. This method may be employed specially on unhealthy conditions of the partner.

(b) Coitus Interruptus

It is also known as withdrawal method. It is the oldest method of birth control practised by man. In this method the penis is withdrawn from the vagina just before ejaculation (discharge) so that the semen is discharged outside the vagina. At present this method is quite popular and a large number of people throughout the world are using this method.

Advantages

1. No artificial device is required for its use.
2. No cost is involved.
3. This method can be used at any time and at any place.

Disadvantages

1. It may cause disturbance in sexual pleasure in either man or woman or both.
2. It may cause psychological disturbances.
3. Failure rate is very high 10-20% since slightest mistake in time of withdrawing the penis can deposit sperms. Sometimes

spermatozoa may enter in the vagina, although coitus is interrupted through :

(i) Escape of a drop of semen before ejaculation

(ii) Ejaculation in stages

(iii) Ejaculation at or close enough to the external sexual organs of the woman.

(iv) Failure to withdraw the penis in time before ejaculation.

Though withdrawal method has number of disadvantages but even then this method is practised all over the world by a large number of people. Some couples are able to use this method successfully while others may find it difficult to manage.

(c) Rhythm Method (Safe Period)

Rhythm method or safe period method is based on the fact that a woman normally produces one egg-cell every month which is shed during the fertile period which is roughly 10th to 20th day after the onset of menstrual period. If sexual intercourse is avoided during this unsafe period or the days when there is a possibility of meeting the female egg with male sperm then the pregnancy can be avoided. During these unsafe days pregnancy can be avoided if the male sperm is not allowed to enter the vagina by using condom etc.

The egg cell is matured at about the middle of her monthly cycle (mensturation), usually 12 to 16 days before the onset of the next period and can live for almost 2 days. The male seed can remain alive in the female body for at least 3 to 5 days.

On the basis of above assumption the period other than fertile period is considered as safe period from conception point of view. In practice, however, it has been observed that time of ovulation varies in different females, and even from cycle to cycle in the same female. Hence this method is not considered reliable.

A women who wants to use this method should know the length of her previous 6-12 menstrual cycles. The exact days of safe and unsafe period can be calculated by subtracting 18 days from the shortest menstrual cycle which will be the first day of fertile period. If 10 days are subtracted from the longest cycle it will be the last day of the fertile period. For example if a woman's menstrual cycle varies from 26-31 days, the fertile period would be from the 8th day to the 21st day of the menstrual cycle, counting day one as the first day of the menstrual period. There are unsafe periods during which the couple should avoid intercourse if they do not want a pregnancy but if they do want a pregnancy they should have intercourse at this time. Broadly speaking a week before and a week after the menses is considered as safe period. During this period the woman is not fertile because she cannot ovulate.

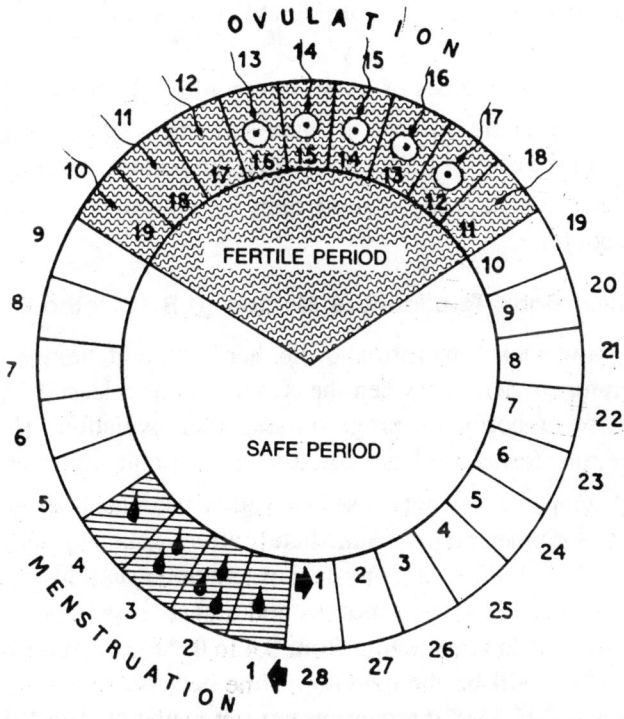

Fig. 3.1 : Safe period method (Rhythm method).

A large number of people throughout the world use rhythm method to avoid pregnancy to take place but it is not considered as a very reliable method.

Advantages

1. No devices are required for its use.
2. No prior medical examination is necessary.

3. No chances of sexual displeasure as other methods create hindrance in one way or the other.

Disadvantages

1. It significantly reduces the number of days for sexual contacts.
2. It is unsuitable for women with irregular periods.
3. Even in safe period women may become pregnant.
4. This method requires considerable self-control and co-operation in a couple.
5. There are chances of errors in recording the menstrual history.
6. It is specially difficult to count safe days during change of life as in the case of menopause when the periods become irregular.
7. This method can be used only by educated and responsible couples.

(d) Basal Body Temperature Method (B.B.T. Method)

During a woman's menstrual cycle, her basal body temperature (the temperature of her body when she is at rest) rises at least 0.4°F because of release of hormone (progesterone) after ovulation. This rise in temperature forms the basis of basal body temperature method.

A woman who want to use this method takes her body temperature with a thermometer daily, immediately after awakening and while still in the bed (i.e. before any physical or emotional activity). The B.B.T. is noted daily for several months and a chart is prepared. The chart will show rise in temperature from 0.4 to 0.8°F on certain days of the cycle which will be the ovulation time because rise in temperature occurs due to release of progesterone after ovulation. Hence fertile and nonfertile periods can be determined. Once the temperature rise is noticed the couple may have intercourse for pregnancy to occur or avoid intercourse for preventing pregnancy to occur.

Advantages

1. It is the natural means of birth control.
2. It does not require artificial means.

Disadvantages

1. It is not reliable method.
2. It cannot be used in ill health.

(e) Cervical Mucus Method (Billings Method)

A woman who wants to use cervical mucus method must learn to recognise the changes which take place in her cervical discharge during her menstrual cycle. During the menstrual cycle, the mucus changes in colour, amount and touch.

After menstrual bleeding ends, most women have one to few days in which no mucus is observed and the vaginal area feels dry. These are called dry days.

After the dry days, a woman begins to see a mucus discharge from her vagina which may be sticky, transparent and watery in nature. When the woman observes any type of mucus before she ovulates, she should realise that ovulation stage is approaching.

It was observed by Billings in 1974 that at the time of ovulation the cervical mucus increases in amount and becomes clear in colour. This mucus feels and looks like raw egg white. These changes are due to the release of hormones–oestrogen and progesterone. The vagina becomes wet so these are called wet days. The last day of wet mucus is called the 'peak day'. These are the fertile days, so couple must not have intercourse during these days to prevent pregnancy. They should not have intercourse for three more days after the wet days or peak day.

After ovulation the cervical mucus becomes sticky and decreases in amount. Her vagina feels dry. This type of mucus does not allow the sperms to enter into the uterus. In some women the vagina remains dry for rest of the menstrual cycle. During these dry days or when the mucus has stopped the couple can have intercourse until next menstrual cycle begins.

Cervical mucus method has main drawbacks that :

1. It requires training of women to identify changes in the cervical mucus.
2. A record is required to be maintained about changes in the cervical mucus.
3. Failure rate is relatively high i.e. about 21%.

(f) Prolonged Lactation Method

This method is also known as lactational amenorrhoea method (L.A.M.) which is based on scientific evidence that women do not become fertile or pregnancy does not take place during full lactational amenorrhoea until her baby is six months old. Full lactation means that the baby is breast fed and no regular supplemental feeding of any type is given to the infant. Amenorrhoea means menstrual bleeding has not resumed.

The mechanisms by which breast feeding delays the return of fertility are not completely understood. But it is observed that ovulation cannot be induced until the harmone (prolactin) level remain high which is secreted by the stimulation of the breasts and nipples of a woman by the infant during suckling. As a result, the regular mensturation is delayed for 11 to 12 months during the period of prolonged lactation.

Studies have shown that the woman who is breast feeding her baby day and night for at least six months from delivery and the menstrual bleeding has not started again, the pregnancy cannot occur in such woman. But the woman who is breast feeding along with supplementary food should know that there are chances for pregnancy to occur. At present about 35 million couples are using this natural method of contraception in the world.

Disadvantages

1. This method provides protection only for 6-10 months after delivery. From 7th month onward it is better to use some other method of contraception in order to avoid risk of pregnancy.
2. The failure rate is high i.e. upto 13%.

(g) Vaginal Washing Method

In this method vagina is immediately washed after intercourse to flush out all sperms. For washing, usually plain water mixed with vinegar, alum, salt or soap is used.

This method is rarely used as a contraceptive method because the failure rate is relatively high i.e. 20-40%.

2. SPACING METHODS

There are a large number of methods which can be used for keeping a space in the birth of children. These methods provide effective protection against pregnancy during the period in which they are used.

(I) BARRIER CONTRACEPTIVES (MECHANICAL METHOD)

Barrier contraceptive or mechanical methods are used either to physically block the union of sperms and ovum or chemically inactivate the sperms in the vagina. The popularity of barrier methods is increasing day by day because these methods are effective and can prevent sexually transmitted diseases and cause no serious adverse effects. The barrier contraceptives are discussed as follows :

(a) Condom (Nirodh)

Condom is made up of very thin sheath of rubber latex or silicon which can be stretched according to size of the erect penis. It is used by the

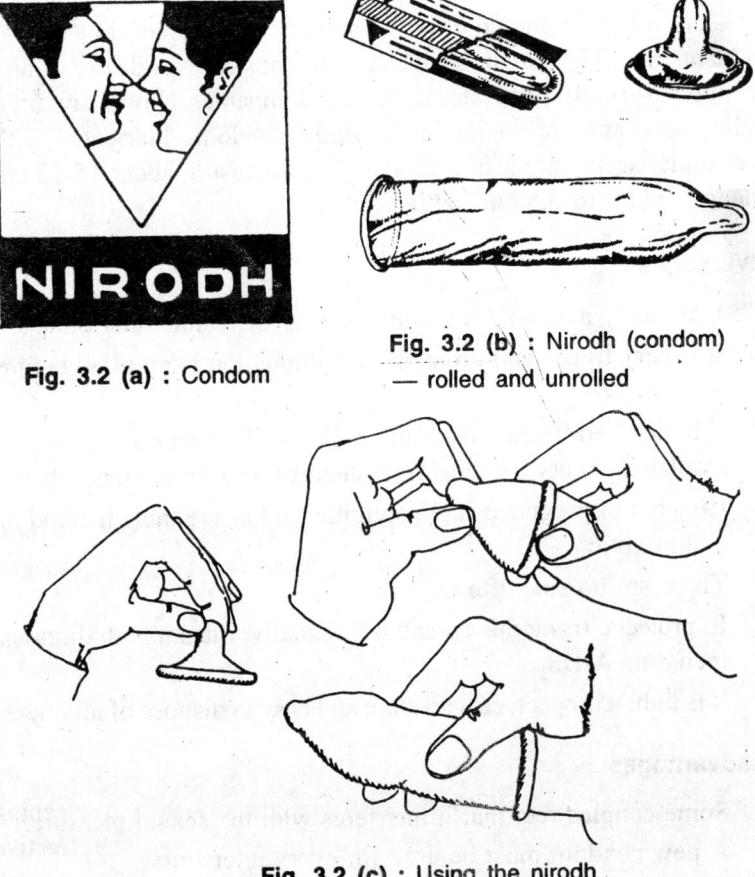

Fig. 3.2 (a) : Condom

Fig. 3.2 (b) : Nirodh (condom)
— rolled and unrolled

Fig. 3.2 (c) : Using the nirodh

man during sex. It is one of the oldest and widely used methods of contraception.

The condom is unrolled on the erect penis before sexual intercourse (and not just before ejaculation, because there are chances that sperms may be present in the pre-coital secretion). While unrolling the Nirodh on the penis, a little space should be left at the end so that the discharged fluid can spill into it. As the Nirodh covers the penis, the sperms cannot go inside the body of the woman, thus acts as barrier.

Sometimes condoms are used along with a spermicidal (cream, jelly or foam tablets placed in the vagina before intercourse) which gives extra protection from pregnancy to occur. Condom provides reliable protection not only from pregnancy but also against sexually transmitted diseases.

A new Nirodh should be used for every intercourse and it should not be re-used. They are available in different shapes and colours and are supplied at subsidised rates by various companies. Now a days high quality condoms are available. Recently condoms lubricated with spermicidal agents are also available. They measure about 15-20 cm in length and 3 to 3.5 cm in diameter.

Advantages

1. It is easily available through a variety of commercial outlets.
2. It is easy to use and no medical examination is required before its use.
3. It is supplied free of cost at all family welfare centres and is also available at very low cost from chemist, grocer and paan shops.
4. Chances of pregnancy are negligible and is a reliable method of contraception.
5. There are no side effects.
6. It protects from the spread of sexually transmitted diseases including AIDS.
7. It is light, compact, easy to store and easy to dispose of after use.

Disadvantages

1. Some couples feel that it interferes with the sexual pleasure.
2. A new condom must be used for every intercourse.
3. It may slip off or tear (rarely) during coitus.

4. In rare cases an individual may be sensitive to rubber.
5. The failure rate is about 14%.

Instructions for the use of Condoms

1. A new condom must be used for every intercourse.
2. It must be fitted on the erect penis before intercourse.
3. The condom must be held carefully when taking the penis out of the vagina after intercourse so as to prevent the spillage of seminal fluid into the vagina.
4. The used condom should not be thrown indiscriminately but it should be wrapped in paper and thrown in the dustbin.

(b) Diaphragm

Vaginal diaphragm is a dome-shaped device made up of soft rubber or latex and fitted with a spring in its rim. It acts as a mechanical barrier because it does not allow the sperms to enter into the uterus. They vary in size running from 50 to 105 mm but 70-80 mm size is most commonly used. The diaphragm is inserted into the vagina before intercourse where it covers the cervix completely and does not allow the sperms to enter into the uterus. It must remain in place at least for six hours after intercourse. To make it more effective a spermicidal cream or jelly should be applied to the diaphragm before use. After use it should be removed from the vagina carefully, washed with soap and water, lubricated with talcum powder and then kept in a good container. It should be periodically replaced with new one because of wear and tear.

Since the diaphragm is to be fitted into the vagina therefore medical advice is necessary for the selection of proper size of diaphragm as well as method of use and method of removal after use.

Advantages

1. It does not interfere with sexual pleasure.
2. It does not hurt or affect either man or woman.
3. It can be placed in the vagina at any time by the woman herself once she learns how to use it.
4. It is comparatively cheap.

Disadvantages and Precautions

1. A doctor or nurse is required to determine the proper size and to give training for its proper use.
2. One size does not fit to all women.
3. Privacy is required for its insertion into the vagina.
4. It is difficult to educate the illiterate women how to use the diaphragm.
5. It must be left in place for at least 6 hours after intercourse.
6. After use it must be thoroughly washed, dried and stored for further use. If proper hygiene is not maintained it may be a source of infection.
7. It must be checked each time before use to exclude defects.
8. Preferably it should be used along with a spermicidal cream or jelly.
9. It must be examined once in a year to see if the prescribed diaphragm is still of the correct size.

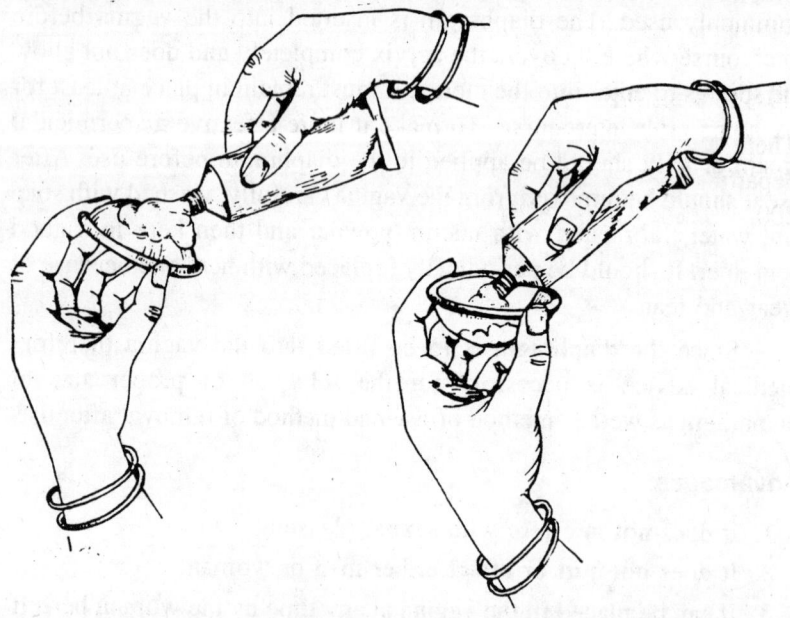

Fig. 3.3 : Diaphragm & Jelly.

(c) Intrauterine Devices (IUDs)

Intrautrine device means inside the uterus. It is inserted into the uterus to prevent conception. There are many types of intrauterine devices but Lippes loop and copper-T are most commonly used in India. If a woman has already borne a child then copper-T is one of the most reliable methods for keeping a desired space in between the existing and the next child.

(i) *Lippes Loop*

It is simply called 'loop' which is a small double 'S' shaped device made of polyethylene. These devices are attached with soft nylon threads so that loop can be removed easily as and when desired. The loop contains a small amount of barium so that it could be seen on X-Ray. The loops are available in different sizes but 27.5 mm length size is most commonly used. The doctor or trained nurse gently places this device in the woman's womb with the help of insertion tube. Previously Lippes loop was very widely used but now it is replaced by copper-T.

(ii) *Copper-T*

There are many types of copper releasing IUDs but in India the department of family welfare has recommended the use of copper-T 200.

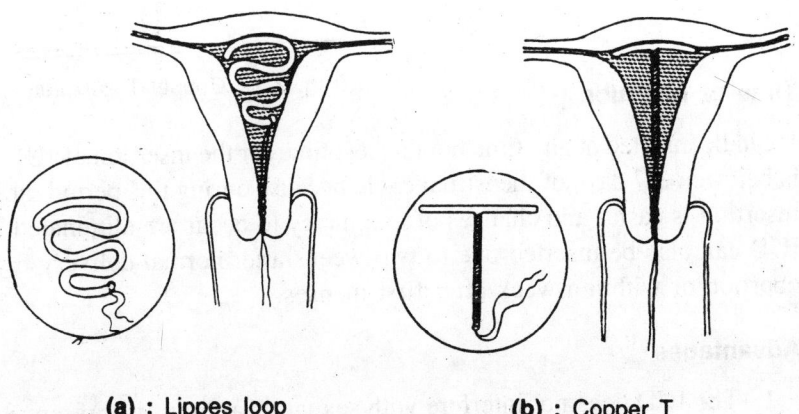

(a) : Lippes loop   (b) : Copper T

Fig. 3.4 (a & b) : Loop & Copper-T

Copper-T is made of polythene and a copper wire is wrapped around the stem of the device which enhances its contraceptive effect. Tail of nylon thread is attached to these devices so that IUD can be easily removed as and when pregnancy is desired. The tail is soft and causes no discomfort to male. The tail can be felt with a finger which assures that IUD is in place.

After thorough examination the copper-T is inserted in the uterus by a doctor or trained nurse. When inside the uterus it does not interfere with the sex life of the wearer. The device can remain in place for a number of years but since copper can dissolve slowly, the copper-T device may be replaced every 3 to 5 years.

Copper-T is available in ready to use pre-packaged sterile disposable units consisting of copper-T, inserter tube with its movable flange and plunger. There is no need to sterilise again.

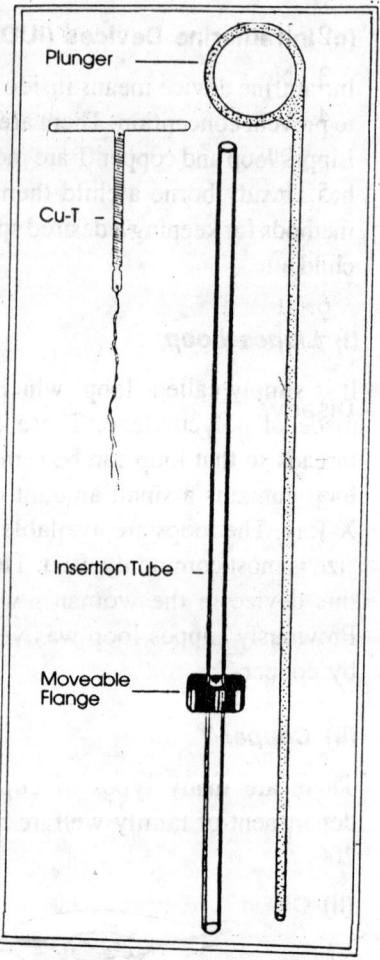

Fig. 3.5 : Copper-T 200 set.

Time of Insertion

It can be inserted at any time but the best time for the insertion of IUD is between 3-7 days of menstrual cycle because during this period the insertion is easier and chances of pregnancy to occur are eliminated. IUD can also be inserted one to two weeks after normal delivery or abortion or within a week after first menses.

Advantages

1. The IUD does not interfere with sexual pleasure as its presence is not felt either by male or female partner during intercourse.

2. It is safe and cheap.

3. No hospitalisation is required.

4. It is a reversible method and can be easily removed by pulling out the tail attached to the IUD.

5. It provides protection from fear of pregnancy for a considerably longer period of time (at least for one year) and requires no attention after insertion.

6. It is a reliable method for spacing birth of the children.

7. Its failure rate is quite low (about 2-3%).

Disadvantages

1. It may be painful when inserted or removed.

2. It may be automatically expelled.

3. Various side effects may be induced like backache, pain in the lower abdomen, discomfort, increased bleeding, cervical perforation, pelvic inflammation etc. These complaints will disappear after a few days or weeks but if these side effects persist for a long time then woman should immediately contact the doctor in order to remove the IUD.

4. The device must be changed at least once every three years.

5. It cannot be used in certain gynaecological problems and pregnancy.

(II) CHEMICAL METHODS

The main object of using the chemical contraceptives is to stop the progress of sperms completely or kill them before they enter into the uterus. Various chemical contraceptives include :

(a) Foam Tablets

These are the tablets which contain spermicidal agent and are inserted deep in the vagina after moistening with water, just 5-10 minutes before the intercourse. The tablets will come in contact with moisture present in the vagina and produce a thick foam which will reduce the mobility of sperms and kill the sperms. Thus they act as physical barrier as well as spermicidal agent. Foam tablets are more effective when they are used along with condoms.

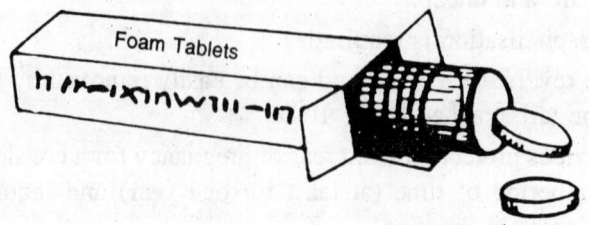

Fig. 3.6 : Foam tablets.

Advantages

1. They are easy to use.
2. They do not interfere with sexual pleasure.
3. Usually there are no side effects.
4. No prior medical examination is necessary.
5. They are good for a woman who has intercourse once a while.

Disadvantages

1. It is not an effective contraceptive method but more effective when used along with a condom.
2. Sometimes side effects like irritation or burning sensation occurs in the vagina.
3. They will have to be inserted 5-10 minutes before intercourse.
4. Deterioration takes place if they are not stored properly.

(b) Contraceptive Creams and Jellies

These are chemical contraceptives which are introduced into the vagina with the help of an applicator. They are applied in sufficient quantity just before intercourse. At body temperature they melt and spread in the vagina and provide a thin film of a chemical barrier. This chemical barrier destroys the sperms. Now-a-days aerosol foam is more commonly used because it is easy to use and more effective. On pressing the actuator the cream is forced into the vagina where it forms a foam.

These creams, jellies or aerosol foams are more effective when they are used in combination with mechanical contraceptives (e.g. condom or diaphragm). When used alone they will be less effective.

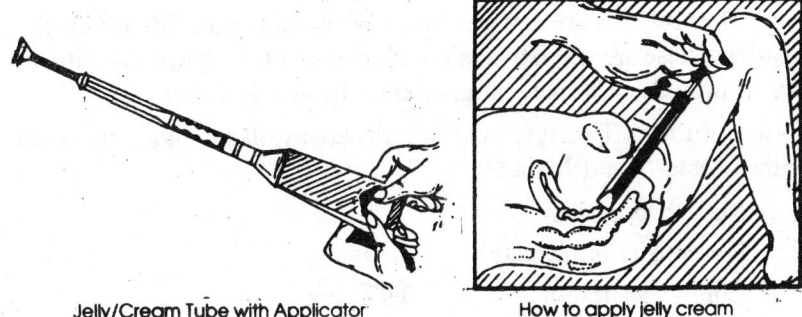

Jelly/Cream Tube with Applicator   How to apply jelly cream

Fig. 3.7 : Creams & jellies.

Advantages

1. It is easy to use.
2. No prior medical examination is necessary.
3. They prove more effective when used along with Nirodh or diaphragm.

Disadvantages

1. When used alone they may not be very effective.
2. They can prove ineffective if used in insufficient quantity.
3. If one hour is lapsed from the time of application to the time of intercourse, there may be a risk of pregnancy.
4. Side effects may include local irritation or soreness in either the man or the woman.

(d) Soluble Tablets (pessaries)

These tablets contain spermicidal agents. They are inserted manually high up in the vagina 5 minutes before intercourse. At body temperature the tablet will melt and form a solution which will release the spermicidal agent on the mouth of the uterus.

(e) Oral Contraceptives (oral pills)

Oral contraceptives are popularly known as 'oral pills' which contain a small amount of an oestrogen and a progesterone. They are one of the most effective and reversible methods of contraception and are particularly suitable for young couples below the age of 30 years.

The oral pills prevent pregnancy by inhibiting ovulation from the ovaries. These are taken by mouth. If an oral pill is taken daily without fail, it provides 100 percent protection from pregnancy.

Types of Pills : Two types of oral pills are available under the brand names Mala-N and Mala-D.

(a) Mala-N contains

Norethisterone acetate	1.0	mg.
Ethinyl oestradiol	0.03	mg.

(b) Mala-D contains

D-norgestrol	0.5	mg.
Ethinyl oestradiol	0.03	mg.

These pills are available in the market and are also supplied free of cost by the government under family welfare programme. Each packet of contraceptive pills contains 28 pills out of which one pill is to be taken daily starting from 4th/5th day of menstruation for 21 days. The remaining 7 pills contain iron which is helpful in checking anaemia.

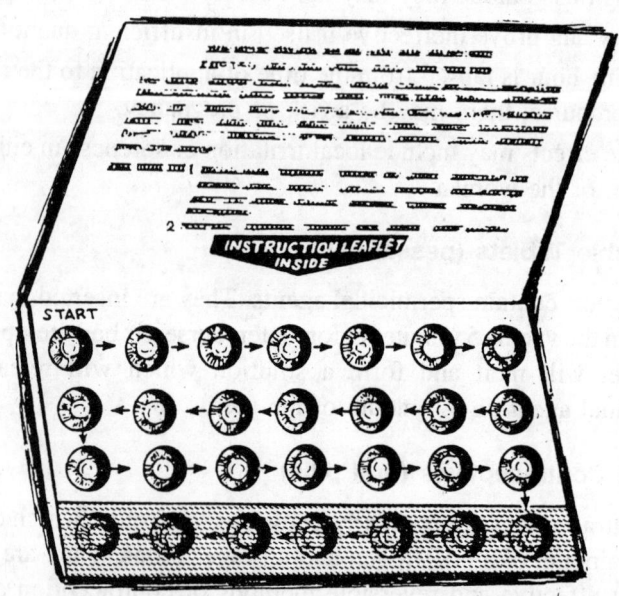

Fig. 3.8 : Mala-D.

When this packet is finished, a new packet must be started from the very next day. It is advisable that an extra packet is always kept handy, so that next cycle of pills can be started without break. This regularity is the most important aspect which ensures high efficacy of the method. A pill should be taken daily at a fixed time, preferably at bed time. However if the woman forgets to take the pill on any particular day, she should take the missed pill as soon as possible or two pills on the next day, one in the morning and another in the evening. If missed on more than a couple of occasions, it should not be discontinued, but another method of contraception like Nirodh should be used along with oral pills upto the date of next menstrual cycle.

Advantages

1. If taken regularly, it is 100% effective.
2. It does not interfere with sexual pleasure.
3. Whenever pregnancy is desired, the pill can be discontinued.
4. It is quite useful for a newly married woman who desires to postpone the birth of her first child.
5. The pill has a number of health benefits like easing menstrual problems and correcting irregular bleeding etc.

Disadvantages

1. A careful history and prior medical examination is necessary before starting the pills.
2. Side effects like dizziness, nausea, headache, vomiting, increase in weight, bleeding between menstrual periods and tenderness of breast are noticed. These symptoms are similar to those of early pregnancy and will disappear after the regular use of pills for 2-3 months. In any case woman must get herself examined medically within 3 months of taking the pills.
3. It requires strong motivation and self discipline for taking the pill daily.

Contraindications

The pill should not be taken in case the woman is
    (i) Pregnant.

(ii) Over 35 years of age.

(iii) Diabetic or there is a history of diabetes in her family or if she is having high blood pressure, chronic liver disease or cancer of the breast or genitals.

(iv) A nursing mother during the first 12 months.

B. PERMANENT METHODS

The contraceptive methods already discussed offer a wide choice for the couples who want to delay the first child or to ensure a minimum gap between two children. Once the family is complete, it is useful to consider the permanent methods which will put an end to the need for contraceptives.

Once the couple decides not to have any further child, sterilization provides permanent protection from pregnancy freeing the couple to enjoy married life without any fear of pregnancy to occur. Adopting a permanent method is a safe and wise step. Either husband or wife can undergo the simple operation for sterilization. In view of its safety and effectiveness the government offers various kinds of incentives in cash and kind to the people who undergo sterilization operations. In males it is known as vasectomy and in females it is known as tubectomy.

(a) Vasectomy

Vasectomy is done in males who do not want more children. It is a simple operation and requires no hospitalisation of the patient because the operation requires hardly 15-20 minutes.

This operation is done under local anaesthesia during which a small cut equal to the size of a grain of wheat is given on both sides of man's scrotum i.e. on each side of the two tubes (vas deferens) which carry the seeds (sperms) from the testes. The cut ends are tied up. This prevents the flow of male seeds into the semen. Thus meeting of male seeds and woman's egg is stopped. So, no pregnancy can take place.

The man's glands are not touched. He continues to enjoy sex as before. He also continues to ejaculate during sex but now his semen does not contain sperms or those seeds which cause pregnancy. There is no difference in his strength or virility (sexual strength).

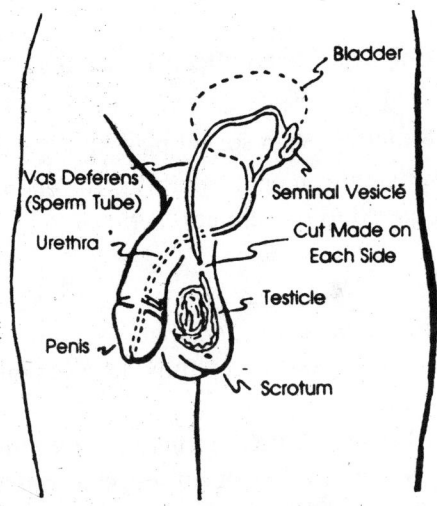

Fig. 3.9 : Vasectomy.

Immediately after the operation the man can go home but preferably he should be kept under observation for at least 2 hours for any signs of shock. Before he leaves for home the dressings should be examined for any untoward bleeding. If there is any bleeding that must be controlled before he leaves for home.

Advice to the Patient of Vasectomy

1. He should not soil the dressings with urine or faeces.
2. He should protect the dressings from wetting during bathing.
3. He should not scratch the operated area even if it itches.
4. He should come to the hospital on 5th day for check up and for removal of stitches.
5. He should not do any hard manual labour or cycling for about one week.
6. He should not have sexual intercourse for about a week. Thereafter he should use Nirodh or abstain from sexual intercourse for three months as a precaution against conception.
7. After three months his semen should be got examined to make sure that there are no sperms present. If no sperms are found then there is no need to use any contraceptive in future.

Advantages

1. It is very simple, safe and effective method of contraception.
2. It does not require hospitalization.
3. It does not interfere with sexual pleasure.
4. After the initial three months following the operation, no further action is required to prevent conception.

Disadvantages

1. It is an irreversible method but in some cases surgical recanalisation has been successfully done but this is not always successful.
2. Nirodh will have to be used during the first three months after the operation or until the semen test confirms the absence of sperms.

(b) Tubectomy

As stated earlier tubectomy is a permanent method of family planning which is done in females. Tubectomy should be done only when the couples are absolutely sure that they do not want more children.

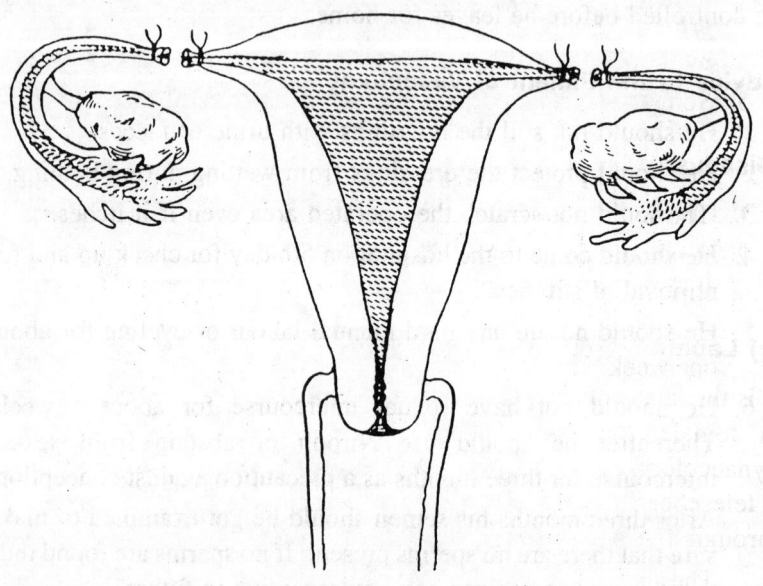

Fig. 3.10 : Tubectomy.

This operation is done under general or spinal anaesthesia during which a small piece of each fallopian tube is removed by giving a small cut. The cut ends are tied so as to block the passage of egg cell. In this way the egg cell won't be able to meet the sperms during sexual intercourse hence no pregnancy can take place.

Hospitalisation is required for 5 to 7 days. After tubectomy, she can do light household work after about 10 days and can resume sexual intercourse after about one month. Tubectomy is considered as a major operation.

Advantages

1. Since it is a permanent method so after the operation, no further action is required by either man or woman for preventing conception.
2. The operation can be done immediately after delivery or abortion in a hospital or at any other time convenient to the woman.
3. There are no side effects or complications when performed by a competent surgeon.
4. The operation is done free of charge in a government hospital, primary health centre or in the family welfare camps organised by the family welfare department.
5. Some cash or kind incentives are given by the government.

Disadvantages

1. The woman will have to stay in the hospital for about 7 days.
2. It is an irreversible method, can be reversed by canalisation but this is not always successful.

(c) Laparoscopy

It is the latest and very sophisticated method of family planning used in females. It is carried out by a team of trained surgeons/gynaecologists with a specialised instrument called 'laparoscope'. It is a telescope like instrument which is introduced into the abdomen through a very small opening.

The abdomen is first inflated with gas (carbon monoxide, nitrogen or air) to push away the intestines from the site of operation. One or

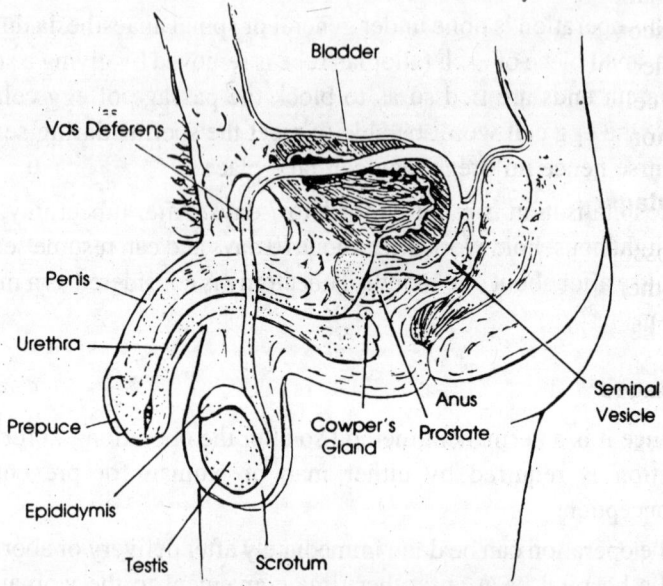

Fig. 3.11 : Male reproductive organs.

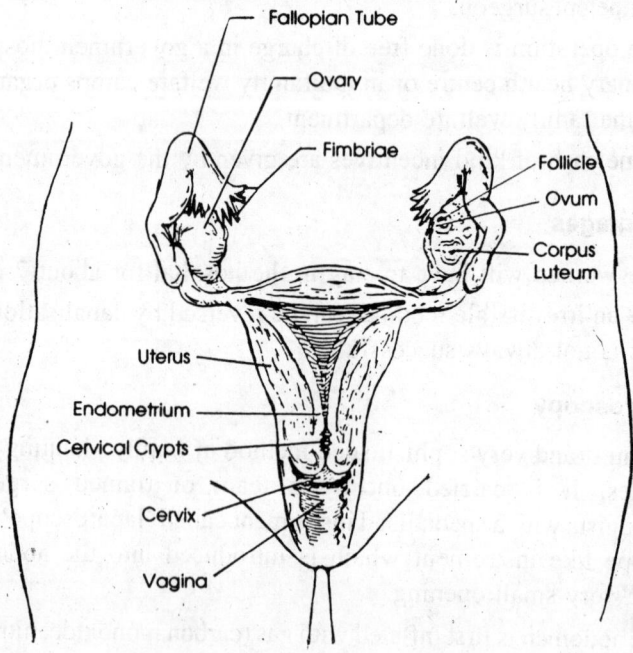

Fig. 3.12 : Female reproductive organs.

two small cuts are made in the lower abdomen. With the help of laparoscope the fallopian tubes are identified. Once the tubes are identified the Falope rings (or clips) are applied to block the passage of egg cell. The Falope rings offer better scope for reversing the tubal occlusion (blockage) later, if necessary.

Advantages

Laparoscopic method of tubectomy has gained considerable popularity over other methods of female sterilization that :

1. The incision made in the abdomen is very small as compared to open operations where large cuts from 5 to 10 inches or more are made so that the surgeon's hand can pass through easily.

2. In spite of tiny incision, the doctor's view of the area is not limited but a magnified picture is flashed on to the T.V. screen which is better than the view obtained during conventional surgery.

3. The small opening causes less injury during and after the operation. Moreover the chances of bleeding and other complications are minimum.

4. A small cut causes less pain afterwards and heals very quickly.

5. Chances of post-operative infections are minimum since the internal organs are not exposed to bacteria.

6. Internal organs are not damaged because they are not pulled out to provide access to the chosen area.

7. One of the biggest advantages is the total time of the doctor as well as patient saved because in this method the patient is hospitalized for one day only. Hence overall cost of operation is decreased.

Disadvantages

1. The instrument is very costly so small hospitals cannot afford to purchase it.

2. In some cases laparoscopic operation may take longer time.

The operations which can be done with a laparoscope are tubectomy, removal of gall bladder with or without stones; removal of appendix, a diseased kidney or lung; hepatic ulcer, hernias and disorders of large intestines.

(C) MEDICAL TERMINATION OF PREGNANCY (MTP)

Abortion

Abortion is defined as the expulsion or removal of an embryo or foetus from the womb at a stage of pregnancy when it is incapable of independent survival (i.e. at any time between conception and 28th week of pregnancy).

Millions of women, married and unmarried specially living in villages die needlessly from the results of illegal abortions performed on them by quacks and untrained persons, often under insanitary conditions. Under desparate conditions the women had induced abortions done from quacks and usually had to pay exorbitant fees which they could ill afford. Due to unskilled efforts and dirty apparatus used many serious complications used to arise and sometimes even led to death of women undergoing illegal abortions.

Medical Termination of Pregnancy Act

To save the lives of millions of women from the hands of quacks doing induced abortions, in 1971, an Act was introduced known as the Medical Termination of Pregnancy Act (1971). According to this Act abortions have been legalised which can be done by a qualified doctor under certain conditions. Wide publicity to this Act should be given in villages so that the women no longer resort to unsafe, illegal means in order to terminate an unwanted pregnancy.

Medical termination of pregnancy should not be considered as a method of family planning. Repeated termination of pregnancy is harmful to the woman. However if pregnancy occurs due to failure of contraceptive methods then the woman can get the pregnancy terminated before 12 weeks of pregnancy under Medical Termination of Pregnancy Act (1971) :

Conditions under which a pregnancy can be terminated under the M.T.P. Act :

1. To save the life of the woman when there is danger to her life due to pregnancy.
2. To prevent grave injury to the physical or mental health of the mother.
3. On humanitarian grounds where the pregnancy has occured due to rape.

4. Where there is a substantial reason to believe that the child to be born would suffer from physical or mental abnormalities.
5. If there is a fear that the environment or the circumstances (social or economical) of the pregnant woman may cause injury to her health.
6. When the pregnancy occurs due to failure of contraceptive method.

M.T.P. should be done as early in pregnancy as possible by a qualified doctor in a hospital or at such places which have the necessary equipment and facilities for termination of pregnancy under safe and hygienic conditions and which have been approved for the purpose by the government.

Usually there are no complications after MTP but sometimes there may be fever or menstrual disturbances. In all such cases the doctor must be consulted immediately.

If pregnancy is to be terminated then it must be terminated as early as possible and before 12 weeks are over. It must be done by trained doctors and the woman should not fall in the hands of quacks and untrained *dais* who may spoil the case and the life of the woman may be in danger.

4

FIRST AID

First aid is defined as the immediate treatment given to the accident victim or sudden illness, quickly and correctly before medical help is made available.

As a result of ever increasing population and complexities of day-to-day routine life, the chances of a person to meet with accidental injuries are increasing. Anything that happens unexpectedly and by chance, affecting health of a person can be called as an accident. Accidents can occur at any time and at any place, usually at odd times and at odd places where a doctor is not generally available. The severity of accident may vary from skin abrasions which may be associated with increased heart beating due to fear upto sudden death of the patient. The accidents require immediate attention and prompt treatment. If the person does not get medical help in time the condition may get worse and his life may be in danger. In such cases the first aid is the kind of treatment which is given to the victim till the medical aid by a doctor is available. First aid is only the first step in treating an injured person in case of accident or sudden illness. It does not mean a complete care and cure of the injuries. After first aid the victim must be taken to a doctor or a hospital.

Objects of First Aid

1. To prevent any danger to life.
2. To prevent further injury and deterioration of the condition of the patient.

3. To give relief from pain.

4. To make medical care available at the earliest.

The first aid can be given by any person who has got training or has been taught the underlying principles of first aid. The first aider should have the following qualities :

1. He should remain as calm and cool as possible.

2. He must be alert and note down the causes and signs of injury.

3. He should be tactful to gain confidence of the patient as well as the persons standing nearby.

4. He should be able to control the crowd and take help from onlookers.

5. He should have self-confidence and must be polite with the patient as well as his attendants.

6. He should have sufficient knowledge to gauge (judge) that out of several injuries which are to be treated first.

7. He should look around for help and send someone to inform the doctor and arrange for ambulance if need arises while he himself should remain with the patient to take his care.

8. In case of serious accident he should immediately inform the nearby police.

Principles of First Aid

1. Reach the site of accident as early as possible because the saving of life may depend on the promptness of action.

2. Take first aid material along with you if it is easily available.

3. Do not waste time asking unnecessary questions.

4. Find out the cause of injury.

5. Immediately separate the victim from the cause of accident e.g. fire, electrical current, falling building, poisonous insects etc. and remove him to a safe place.

6. Find out whether the patient is conscious or unconscious, dead or alive.

7. Decide the priority of giving first aid measures e.g. restoration of cardiac functions, restoration of breathing, stoppage of bleeding etc.

8. Arrange for medical help.
9. Keep the patient warm and comfortable as far as possible.
10. If the patient is conscious, give encouragement and reassure him that he is alright.
11. If any specific equipment is not available try to improvise it.

First Aid Kit

A small portable first aid kit should be available in every home, schools, colleges, buses, factories, swimming pools and at other public places. The kit should be handy and should contain at least the following articles:

(i) Sterile gauge
(ii) Bandages of different sizes
(iii) Triangular bandages
(iv) Adhesive bandages
(v) A pair of scissors and forceps
(vi) Aromatic spirit of ammonia
(vii) Antiseptic solution like dettol, mercurochrome etc.
(viii) Burn ointments
(ix) Emergency drugs like pain killers, antibiotics and packets of O.R.S. etc.

All these articles should be properly arranged and well preserved in the kit so as to prevent contamination or spoilage. These items should be periodically examined. Spoiled or contaminated articles as well as expired medicines should be replaced with new ones. The first aid kit should be kept handy and in ready to use form because emergency may arise at any time.

Type of First Aid

Accidents may occur at any time and at any place like at home, on roads, in factories or as a result of natural calamities, burns, electric shock, drowning, insect bite and snake bite etc. The first aider may not be always present at the site of accident but as soon as he comes to know about the accident, he must reach immediately at the site of accident. On reaching there he may obtain a brief history of accident either from the patient himself if he is conscious or from the onlookers if the patient is unconscious. If the patient is conscious and able to give reliable information, examine first at the points where there is pain or obvious signs and symptoms indicating injury or illness. The patient should then be examined for :

(i) **Pulse Rate** : If the pulse is felt, it indicates that the patient is alive but if the pulse is not felt even after external cardiac massage, it means patient is dead. If the pulse is very weak and rapid it indicates severe bleeding, external or internal.

(ii) **Breathing** : Check the breathing. Is it absent,slow or fast? If the patient requires breathing, give him artificial respiration.

(iii) **Pallor** : Note the pallor or degree of whiteness of the tongue, conjunctiva and nails. It will indicate the severity of bleeding.

(iv) **Colour of Tongue and Lips** : If the colour of tongue and lips has turned blue it indicates that there is lack of oxygen.

(v) **Bleeding** : The body parts like ears, mouth, nose and other parts must be checked for bleeding. If there is severe bleeding that must be checked immediately.

(vi) **Fracture** : The movement of joints should be checked to see if there is any fracture or not.

(vii) **Burns** : The cause and degree of burns should be noted.

(viii) **Poisons** : The patient must be examined to ensure whether he has taken any poison or not which can be determined by noting the signs and symptoms of poisonous materials.

After noting the brief history of the accident, promt first aid must be given. Delay at any stage may lead to death of the patient.

1. ACCIDENTS

Anything that happens unexpectedly and by chance which affects the health of a person can be called as an accident. Accident can happen at any time and at any place the intensity of which may vary from minor skin abrasions upto sudden death of the victim.

Accidents do not just happen, they are caused. Many of the accidents are the results of carelessness, thoughtlessness, neglect and momentary lack of concentration on the part of human beings. Many of the accidents are caused due to tiredness, stress, worry, anger, illness, bad news or even good news. Drinking of alcohol also leads to many kinds of accidents. It is not always that the person who causes accident suffers but the innocent person may suffer more.

With the increase in population, rapid growth of industrialization and urbanization the way of life has become very fast which is the basic cause of fatal accidents and has become one of the major causes of death. The accidents can be classified as follows :

1. Indoor accidents
2. Outdoor accidents
3. Accidental poisoning
4. Seasonal accidents

1. Indoor Accidents

Indoor accidents can happen :

(a) In the kitchen where gas stoves, electrically operated kitchen wares, pressure cookers, knives etc. are used.

(b) In the bathrooms where electric geysers, washing machines and acid bottles for cleaning purposes are stored.

(c) In the sitting rooms, dining rooms, stair case etc. due to slipperiness, inadequate light and haphazard arrangement of the luggage.

(d) In homes the accidents due to children of pre-school age and elderly persons are very common. The accidents which occur due to children include falls, accidental poisoning, swallowing of foreign bodies, putting foreign bodies in the ear, nose or wind pipe; burns while playing with fire or due to accidents in the kitchen; electric shock while playing with faulty electrical appliances.

2. Outdoor Accidents

(a) Now a days road accidents have become a great nuisance not only in big cities but everywhere due to increase in vehicular traffic, rash driving and lack of traffic rules. A large number of deaths occur daily due to road accidents.

(b) Industrial accidents : Persons who work on the machines generally fall prey to accidents, often very serious.

(c) Accidents in the sports grounds.

(d) Accidents in the sea, river, well, lakes and swimming pools etc.

3. Accidental Poisoning

Poisoning may take place either accidentally such as food poisoning; in children due to carelessness of the parents or intentionally to commit suicide.

4. Seasonal Accidents

According to season a number of accidents take place e.g. in summer season cases of heat stroke and during extreme winter cases of chilblain. A number of fire accidents occur during Diwali. Similarly a number of different kinds of accidents occur during melas and other festival seasons.

First Aid in Accidents

   (i) Redirect the traffic if necessary.
  (ii) Do not allow anybody to smoke because it may cause fire or explosion if petrol has spilled due to accident.
 (iii) If bleeding is there control it immediately by direct pressure on the affected area.
  (iv) If heart beat or breathing is not proper try to revive it.
   (v) Get aside the crowd tactfully so as to arrange proper ventilation.
  (vi) If the victim is mentally shocked give him assurance and keep him in a cool and calm mental level.
 (vii) If the victim is unconscious, place him in the recovery position.
(viii) Call for the doctor or arrange an ambulance.
  (ix) Keep the injured person's mouth and nose free from obstruction by vomits in order to avoid chocking of wind pipe.
   (x) If the person is unconscious do not give him anything to drink, not even water. It may cause chocking of wind pipe, moreover it may cause obstruction if immediate operation is required to save his life.
  (xi) If fracture is there do not move fractured part unless necessary.

(xii) Keep the body of the injured person warm by covering it with blankets.

(xiii) Take the injured person to the hospital as early as possible.

2. ABRASIONS

Abrasion is an injury caused to the skin by forceful rubbing or scraping. During this state there is a possibility of swelling, contamination and infection. The abrations are very painful because the nerve endings are exposed.

First Aid

(i) Clean the wound with antiseptic solution and remove all dirt particles and foreign particles attached to the injured area.

(ii) Apply an antiseptic solution and if necessary apply non-adherent dressing or sterile gauze.

(iii) Give an injection of tetanus toxoid.

3. CUTS (INCISED OPEN WOUNDS)

These are caused by any sharp-edged article like knife, razor, blade, broken glass, sword, axe etc.

First Aid

(i) Stop bleeding by applying pressure.

(ii) Apply antiseptic solution followed by non-adherent or sterile dressing.

4. CHOCKING

Chocking is the condition when air passage is blocked and there is difficulty in breathing. Air passage may be blocked if food or foreign bodies like artificial teeth, coin, seed etc. enters in the wind pipe or water enters into the air passage as in the case of drowning. Chocking is more commonly seen in young children. Death may result due to complete blockage of air passages.

First Aid

(i) Remove the foreign particle by bending the adult over the knees and give a number of blows on his shoulders. In case of child hold him upside down with one hand and with other hand give a number of blows on his shoulders until the foreign particle is thrown out.

(ii) Keep the body warm by light blankets.

5. FOREIGN BODY IN THE THROAT

The foreign bodies which may enter in the throat include coin, marble, seed, peanuts, fish bone etc. The foreign body may irritate the throat and patient feels uncomfortable and complains pain in the throat. The vocal cord muscles are tightened due to which he has difficulty in breathing, talking and swallowing.

First Aid

(i) Reassure the patient.

(ii) Make the patient sit in a comfortable position with mouth downward. Give a few blows on his shoulders until the foreign body is thrown out.

(iii) If the object does not come out, give him cooked potatoes, banana, soft rice or soft bread to eat. It will help the swallowed object to pass down.

(iv) Do not give purgatives.

(v) Examine stools on next morning for the foreign body.

6. FOREIGN BODY IN THE EAR

Children may push foreign bodies like peas, grams, beads, buttons, pieces of stones or pieces of chalk etc. into their ears. An insect may also enter into the ear, if not removed may cause serious complications.

First Aid

(i) Put warm oil in the ear to float out the insect.

(ii) If unsuccessful then contact the doctor.

(iii) Under no circumstances try to remove foreign body with a match stick, tweezers or hair pins etc. During this act the delicate membrane called the ear drum may be damaged.

7. FOREIGN BODY IN THE NOSE

Children may push foreign bodies like peas, grams, buttons, pieces of stones or small coins into their nose. The patient feels uncomfortable and complains of pain and irritation in the nose. There may be bleeding if sharp object like pin, nail, needle or broken glass has been pushed into the nose.

First Aid

(i) Make the patient sneeze by using snuff or entering the end of a piece of thread in the opposite nostril. The foreign body may be expelled by sneezing.

(ii) If unsuccessful seek the help of a doctor.

(iii) Do not try to remove it with a pin or a hook.

8. FOREIGN BODY IN THE EYE

Often small particles of dust, wood, stone, coal, glass or an insect may get into the eyes and cause irritation, redness and watering in the eyes and vision may be blurred.

First Aid

(i) Make the patient sit in a chair.

(ii) Ask him not to rub the eyes.

(iii) Gently wipe the foreign body out with a wisp of cotton wool or with the folded corner of a clean handkerchief.

(iv) Wash the eyes with warm water.

(v) Put eye drops.

(vi) Do not attempt to remove a foreign body lodged in the eye ball.

(vii) If strong acids have entered into the eyes wash it out by washing the eyes with weak solution of sodium carbonate.

(viii) If strong alkalies have entered into the eyes wash it out by washing the eyes with vinegar solution.

(ix) If unsuccessful, take the patient to the doctor.

9. FOREIGN BODY IN THE SKIN

A sharp object like nail. pin, piece of glass or thorn may enter the skin of feet or hands. If a part of the foreign body is projecting out, it is grasped and pulled out. But if it is deep seated and cannot be pulled easily then the patient should be taken to the doctor. After removing the foreign body from the skin, an antiseptic solution like dettol or iodine should be applied to the affected part.

10. SHOCK

Shock is defined as a condition of severe depression of vital functions of the body due to poor circulation of blood. This inadequate blood supply to body organs deprives the tissues from oxygen and other nutrients required by the body to carry out routine metabolic activities. Shock may be due to excessive loss of blood as occurs after internal or external haemorrhage, head injury, chest injury, dehydration due to severe diarrhoea or vomiting, burns, electric shock, poisoning, severe bacterial infection (bacteremic shock), a severe allergic reaction (anaphylactic shock), overdoses with certain drugs like narcotics or barbiturates, or emotional shock due to personal happiness or sadness. Sometimes shock may result from a combination of any of these causes.

Shock is a very serious condition and if not handled promptly and properly may lead to death. So prompt and efficient first aid treatment is of paramount importance.

Types of Shocks

Different types of shocks have already been mentioned in the above paragraph as :

    (i) Haemorrhagic shock

    (ii) Neurogenic shock

    (iii) Anaphylactic shock, and

    (iv) Toxic shock.

But mainly there are two main types of shocks.

    (i) Neurogenic shock (when nerves are involved but there is no blood loss).

    (ii) Haemorrhagic shock (when there is excessive loss of blood due to severe injuries, burns or dehydration).

Signs and Symptoms

The signs and symptoms of shock include dryness of mouth, blueness of lips, paleness of skin, coldness of skin, pupils dialated, vision blurred, anxiety, trembling, difficulty in breathing, fast pulse and temporary loss of consciousness. Blood pressure is generally low, drops of perspiration appear on lips, forehead, palms, soles and armpits. He may be restless or lose alertness. He feels thirsty. Sometimes the patient may seem alert but may suddenly collapse.

Emergency Treatment of Shock

In shock prompt and efficient treatment is required. Failure to do so may lead to death of the patient. Following tips should be observed:

   (i) Remove the patient to a well ventilated area.

  (ii) Remove the crowd tactfully so as to provide proper ventilation and relief of fear and anxiety to the patient.

 (iii) Keep the patient quite in lying down flat position with head lowered and turned to a side. Raise the legs slightly upward by keeping a pillow under the legs so as to improve blood circulation.

 (iv) If there is difficulty in breathing, raise the head and chest of the patient.

  (v) Loosen the clothings but do not remove them.

 (vi) Keep the patient warm with a blanket.

(vii) Do not give either hot or cold drink to the patient because he may require an emergency operation by the doctor.

(viii) Immediately arrange to shift the patient to a hospital.

11. SNAKE BITE

There are about 2500 species of snakes. Out of these only about 200 varieties are poisonous. Poisonous snakes are found all over the world. All sea snakes are poisonous. Most snakes bite only if they are provoked. The bite of all snakes is not poisonous because when the snake bites in its self defence, little or no venom is injected into the body of the victim. Most of the people die not because of venom but from fear and wrong treatment.

In case of snake bite the type of snake must be identified, because if the snake is nonpoisonous there is no need of giving antivenom treatment but if the snake is poisonous antivenom treatment should be given. If the snake cannot be found or cannot be identified, it should be treated as poisonous and general antivenom treatment should be immediately given without wasting much time in search or identification of the snake.

Signs and Symptoms

Signs and symptoms of mild to moderate snake poison include nausea, vomiting, mild swelling and pain at the site of wound, shortness of breath, rapid pulse and dimmed vision. In case of severe poisoning the symptoms include rapid swelling, numbness and pain at the site of wound, blurred vision, shock, convulsions and paralysis. There is loss of consciousness, difficult breathing and slow pulse.

First Aid Treatment

  (i) Lay the patient down, try to cool and calm him. Give him assurance as he is generally very frightened.

 (ii) Do not allow him to move the bitten part because the movement may favour faster absorption of poison into systemic circulation.

(iii) Apply a constricting band, cloth or tourniquet above the fang mark to prevent the spread of poison to other parts of the body through veins and to prevent the flow of blood towards the heart.

 (iv) Wash the wound with soap and water.

  (v) Make a sharp cut (cross wise) over the bitten area and allow to bleed by squeezing the area.

 (vi) Suck out the poison with a suction pump or by mouth (carefully) and spit it out. Be sure that there are no ulcers in the mouth of the sucker.

(vii) If breathing ceases give artificial respiration.

(viii) Transfer the patient immediately to a hospital.

12. TOURNIQUETS

Tourniquets are the devices usually made up of cord, rubber tube, leather or tight bandage which is tied around an arm or leg to prevent the flow of blood or to retard the spread of poison into the blood circulation as in the case of snake bite. Because of its tightness it will not allow the flow of blood beyond the part over which it is tied. Hence there is a risk of permanent damage leading to the occurrence of gangrene, if taurniquet is left in place for more than 15 minutes.

Tourniquets are no longer recommended as a first aid measure to stop bleeding or spread of poison because of the danger of reducing the supply of oxygen to other tissues. However a temporary tourniquet to increase the distention of veins when a sample of blood is being taken is not harmful because here the tourniquet is to be tied only for a very short period.

Burns and Scalds

Burns are the injuries which are caused by dry heat like fire, flames, hot metals, chemicals e.g. strong acids like sulphuric acid, nitric acid, hydrochloric acid; strong alkalies like sodium hydroxide, potassium hydroxide, ammonium hydroxide etc., electricity and radiations.

Scalds are the injuries caused by moist heat like boiling water, steam, hot oil and coal tar, hot wax etc.

Both burns and scalds cause similar damage to the body tissues hence the first aid treatment is similar. The burns may be superficial or deep. The degree of burns varies from minor redness of the affected area (first degree), blisters on the skin of affected area (second degree) upto damage to deeper layers of skin and body tissues (third degree). In third degree burns the base of the burnt tissue looks leathery or dead white. They are most painful type of burns.

The danger from burns depends on the area of burns rather than the degree of burns. Superficial burns over a large area of the body are more dangerous than complete damage or charring of deeper layers of skin and body tissues of a particular part. The most serious consequences of burns is shock. Infection due to contamination is another serious condition that may follow the burns.

First Aid Treatment

    (i) Put off the fire by throwing water, covering the flames with blanket or coat.

(ii) Without wasting time put plenty of cold water or any other non-inflammable liquid over the burnt part. If possible immerse the affected part in cold water for 15-20 minutes or until the pain disappears (In case of extensive burns do not immerse the part for a long time, as it may intensify the shock). If that is not possible, soak clean cloth in cold water and put it over burnt area. It needs to be changed frequently. This treatment with cold water will remove residual heat from tissues and prevent further damage.

(iii) Do not try to remove the clothings from the burnt area rather cut them around.

(iv) Keep the victum calm and in lie down position to avoid shock.

(v) Give him reassurance.

(vi) Do not disturb the blisters in anyway.

(vii) Do not use absorbent cotton, oily substances, antiseptics, flour, butter, baking soda or ink on the burn.

(viii) Remove immediately from the body anything of constricting nature like rings, bangles, belt, boots etc. They may be difficult to remove afterwards as the limbs begin to swell and gangrene may develop.

(ix) Do not touch the burnt area more than absolutely necessary.

(x) Give any liquid to the victim to drink if he is conscious.

(xi) In case of chemical burns, wash the area with water until all chemical has been washed away.

(xii) If eyes are affected with burns, wash them thoroughly and afterwards cover with sterile dressings.

(xiii) If the burning is extensive, wrap the victim in a clean cloth and shift the patient immediately to a nearby hospital.

13. ELECTRIC SHOCK

This happens when a person comes in contact with a defective electrical instrument, live naked electrical wires or devices or atmospheric electricity as in lightening. The extent of tissue damage may vary with the type and strength of current and length of contact etc. In case of D.C. (direct current) shock, the patient remains stuck to the source of electricity until the current is broken, hence the damage is large. In case of A.C. (alternate current) shock, the patient is thrown away from the source of electricity and the damage is less but there may be physical injury. In both cases the damage may vary from a mild injury to severe burns, paralysis of breathing and heart damage. The heat produced during passage of the current through the body causes deep burns. Damp clothing and footwear, damp ground, working on metallic stool which is a good conductor of electricity aggravates the damage.

First Aid Treatment

   (i) Switch off the electric current and remove the plug from the socket.

  (ii) Separate the victim from the source of current with a long wooden stick or any other nonconductor of electricity. If the current is on never try to separate the victim with naked hands or bare-footed.

 (iii) If necessary give artificial respiration and cardiac massage.

 (iv) If need arises shift the patient to a hospital as early as possible.

  (v) Keep his body warm by covering with a blanket.

 (vi) Treat shock if present.

(vii) Treat burns.

14. POISONING

A poison is a substance which when introduced in the body or brought in contact with any part thereof, in sufficient quantity will produce ill health or even death. A poison can be consumed accidentally, for suicidal purpose or may be administered for homicidal purpose.

Some of the poisons include : salts of arsenic, bismuth, mercury, copper, gold, and other heavy metals; phosphorus, chlorine, bromine and iodine; strong acids and alkalies; poisonous fungi; bites of dogs, wild animals, snakes, scorpion, bee, wasp or other insects; plants like datura, nux vomica, aconite etc. The poison may enter into the body by any of the following routes :

 (i) **Oral :** Contaminated food, drugs, alcohol, insecticides, strong acid, strong alkali etc.

(ii) **Inhalation :** Carbon monoxide, carbon dioxide, anaesthetic agents etc.

(iii) **Injection :** Narcotics, sedatives and toxic agents etc.

(iv) **Skin :** Pesticides etc.

(v) **Bites :** Dog, wild animals, snake, bee, wasp etc.

Preventive Measures of Poisoning

Poisoning is a serious matter and if due care is not taken it may lead to death of the victim. So due precautions should be taken while storing poisonous substances to avoid accidental poisoning specially by the children. The following precautions should be taken :

(i) Always keep drugs under lock and key or beyond the reach of the children.

(ii) Do not store medicines for long periods. Expired drugs must be discarded.

(iii) Take proper precautions while storing and handling common poisonous substances like insecticides, pesticides, disinfectants and petroleum products.

(iv) Do not take drugs in the dark.

(v) Always read label of the container while taking the drug.

(vi) Do not put harmful liquids in the bottles of cold drinks. By mistake children may consume it thinking as cold drink.

(vii) Do not burn coal in closed rooms as it produces a highly poisonous gas carbon monoxide.

(viii) Use cooking gas carefully.

(ix) Get your pets immunized against rabies.

(x) Carefully destroy the empty containers of poisonous substances.

(xi) Remove poisonous plants from the premises as well as surroundings.

First Aid Treatment

In poisoning prompt first aid should be given

(i) If the person is conscious, ask him what he has swallowed, in what quantity and at what time ?

(ii) If there are empty containers, wrappers or drugs lying near the patient collect and examine them which will provide information regarding the poison he has consumed. In turn it will help in giving the right treatment.

(iii) If the person is conscious and co-operative, induce vomiting by any of the following methods :

    (a) By tickling the back of patient's throat with the help of fingers.

    (b) By administering a glass of warm water containing two teaspoonful of common salt.

    (c) By administering emetic drug like syrup of ipecac.

The vomited material should be preserved for chemical analysis.

(iv) If the patient is unconscious or is suspected to have consumed strong acid or strong alkali then do not induce vomiting because these are corrosive poisons which burn the mouth, throat and stomach. There is severe pain in throat and abdomen. Breathing is difficult. In such cases give following first aid :

    (a) Do not induce vomiting.

    (b) For strong acids like sulphuric acid, hydrochloric acid etc. give chalk powder, milk of magnesia, calcium hydroxide or sodium bicarbonate (baking powder) in water.

    (c) For strong alkalies like sodium hydroxide, potassium hydroxide, strong ammonia etc. give lemon juice, vinegar or butter milk.

    (d) Apply ghee, oil or glycerin over burnt area in the mouth.

(v) After vomiting and gastric lavage give the patient milk, tea, coffee or egg albumin orally.

(vi) In case of gaseous poisoning like smoke, carbon monoxide and carbon dioxide the following first aid measures should be taken:

    (a) As quickly as possible take the patient out of the room filled with gas, to an open place where fresh air is available.

    (b) Avoid crowding near the patient so as to provide fresh air to him.

    (c) Loosen his clothings.

    (d) If necessary give him artificial respiration.

    (e) If condition is serious immediately shift him to a hospital.

   (vii) If poisoning through skin has occurred wash the affected area with plenty of water and ask the patient to drink as much water as he can.

 (viii) Give specific antidote if specific poison is detected otherwise administer (burnt chopati or charcoal) universal antidote consisting of 2 parts of activated charcoal, 1 part magnesium oxide (milk of magnesia) and 1 part of tannic acid (strong tea).

   (ix) If the symptoms are serious, shift the victim immediately to a hospital emergency room.

    (x) Inform the police.

15. HEART DISEASES

(a) Angina Pectoris

In this condition there is pain in the chest which is induced by exercise and relieved by rest, and may spread to the jaws and arms. Angina pectoris occurs when there is less supply of blood to the heart itself by the coronary arteries. This may be associated with exertion, emotion, exposure to cold or overeating.

First Aid

    (i) Give him complete bed rest.

   (ii) Whenever there is pain keep a tablet of nitroglycerin under his tongue. This will help to dilate the coronary arteries and improve the blood supply.

  (iii) Ask the patient not to indulge in laborious work.

  (iv) Overweight should be reduced.

   (v) In severe cases his bed room should be on the ground floor.

  (vi) If coronary arteries are blocked, bypass surgery may be suggested.

(b) Acute Myocardial Infraction (Heart Attack)

Acute myocardial infraction is also known as heart attack. It is one of the greatest and most important medical emergencies which should be treated promptly otherwise life of the patient may be in danger. In this disease there is damage or death of a part of heart muscles or due to deposition of cholesterol in coronary vessels due to which there is interruption of blood supply to that area of the heart. Myocardial infraction is usually confined to the left ventricle.

Acute myocardial infraction generally occurs to middle-aged and obese persons; persons who take diet rich in fats and cholesterol, habitual drinkers and chronic smokers. The incidence of heart attack is quite high in males as compared to females.

At the time of heart attack there is severe pain in the chest which is radiating to the medial side of the left arm. It usually persists for several hours. There is fall in blood pressure and also shock. The respiration is fast and there is profuse perspiration. Sometimes patient may have vomiting and he feels restless.

First Aid Treatment

  (i) Give him complete bed rest.

 (ii) Give a sublingual tablet of sorbitrate which will dilate the coronary vessels and relieve pain.

   (iii) Loosen clothings of the patient and reassure him.

   (iv) Give an injection of morphine or pethidine to relieve pain.

   (v) If oxygen is available, administer it.

   (vi) If cardioactive drugs e.g. digoxin, lidocaine etc. are available, administer them immediately.

  (vii) Arrange to shift the patient to the hospital emergency room as early as possible.

 (viii) Do not allow the patient to walk to the emergency room but carry him on a stretcher or wheel chair.

16. HAEMORRHAGE

Haemorrhage is defined as the severe loss of blood from the blood vessel(s). Haemorrhage may be external or internal. In external haemorrhage the blood escapes from the external parts of the body. In internal haemorrhage blood passes into the tissues surrounding the ruptured blood vessels. A person may die from internal bleeding even if a small amount of blood remains inside the surrounding tissues. Internal bleeding from the stomach is indicated by vomiting blood, if blood comes out during coughing it means lungs are ruptured, if blood is present in the urine it indicates that urinogenital passage is ruptured and if stools appear jet black, it indicates rupture in the intestines. In such cases medical help should be taken immediately because excessive loss of blood from the body may lead to shock, collapse and death, if bleeding is not checked. Rupture of major blood vessel, such as the temporal artery can lead to a loss of several liters of blood in a few minutes. Therefore it is very important to check bleeding immediately.

First Aid Treatment

(i) Minor bleeding which occurs due to rupture of capillaries during playing or at work will stop automatically after sometime or apply firm pressure and bandage. Afterwards apply some antiseptic solution.

(ii) In case of external bleeding remove the clothings from the affected part.

(iii) Lay the person down in a comfortable position and raise the injured part (if no fracture is suspected).

(iv) Apply direct pressure on the exposed bleeding part using bandages or handkerchief etc. to stop the bleeding. In case of severe bleeding press the ruptured blood vessel against the underlying bone, it may be helpful for quick, temporary and partial control of bleeding until cloth for direct pressure is obtained.

(v) The bandage should not be too tight otherwise it may affect the blood supply to other parts of the body.

(vi) Do not try to control the bleeding of neck and head by applying direct pressure, it may be dangerous.

(vii) Keep the patient warm.

(viii) Check the pulse rate and general health of the patient.

(ix) If the case is unmanageable shift him immediately to the nearby hospital emergency room.

17. FRACTURES

The breakage of bone is known as fracture. Fracture(s) can occur during an accident where bones may break (fracture) or may displace from the joints (dislocation). The fractures are of the following types:

(a) **Simple Fracture (Closed Fracture)** : In simple fracture a bone is broken but there is no break in the skin.

(b) **Compound Fracture (Open Fracture)** : In compound fracture a bone is broken and there is an open wound in the soft tissues and the skin, or sometimes a bone may protrude out through such wound.

Compound fractures are more serious than simple fractures. They usually involve extensive damage to the tissues and may become infected.

(c) **Complicated Fracture** : In complicated fracture there is an injury to blood vessel, nerve or any vital organ like brain, lungs or spleen etc.

Signs and Symptoms

(i) Pain at or near the site of the fracture.

(ii) Tenderness or pain over the affected area, on applying pressure.

(iii) Swelling at the site of the fracture.

(iv) There may be deformity.

(v) The patient is unable to move the affected part.

(vi) Unnatural movements (crepitus or grating) may be felt or heard. When one end of the broken bone moves against the other, a peculiar sound is heard which is known as crepitus.

General First Aid Measures for Any Fracture

(i) Immediately control bleeding by applying pressure bandage.

(ii) Cover all the wounds with sterile dressings.

(iii) Immobilise the fractured part immediately so as to avoid injury to nearby parts of the body by movements of the fractured part which may even pierce the tissues or the skin. For this purpose bandages or splints may be used. Another part of the body can also be used e.g. fractured arm can be fixed to trunk by using slings, a broken leg may be tied to the other leg.

Immobilization of broken bones is important in order to:

(a) Prevent pain.

(b) Prevent further damage to other parts by the broken ends.

(c) Support the tissues which are ordinarily supported by the bones which are now fractured.

(d) Accelerate the rapid healing of the broken bones.

(iv) Do not move fractured part unless necessary.

(v) During immobilization of broken bones use adequate padding in the natural hollows.

(vi) Do not give anything orally to the patient because emergency operation may be required.

(vii) Keep the patient warm.

(viii) Treat the shock, if necessary.

(ix) Analgesics may be given if the patient is having pain.

(x) Arrange to shift the patient to the hospital as early as possible.

18. CARDIO-PULMONARY RESUSCITATION

Generally when people see an unconscious person they try to revive him therefore they put water in his mouth. This is a very wrong practice. Instead of giving relief to the patient it may complicate the problem because the water given by mouth to an unconscious person may go into his lungs and immediate death of the patient may take place due to chocking of respiratory passage. So never give anything orally to an unconscious person. Never keep pillow under his head it may block his breathing. After understanding the emergency and observing all the precautions immediately start CPR (cardio-pulmonary respiration). If respiration and circulation are restored within short period then victim's life can be saved.

Difficulty in breathing may be due to asphyxia. Asphyxia is a condition in which the lungs do not get sufficient air or oxygen due to obstruction or damage to any part of the respiratory system. Brain cells cannot live for more than about four minutes without oxygen. Drowning, electric shock and gas poisoning are the three most common accidents likely to result in asphyxia. Asphyxia may also occur from such accidents as choking, hanging, burial under earth, grains etc. or on entering in burning building. Excessive use of alcohol and drugs may also cause breathing to stop. Respiratory diseases like bronchial asthma, pulmonary tuberculosis etc. may also lead to asphyxia.

CPR or Cardio-Palmonary Resuscitation consists of artificial respiration and artificial circulation. Cardiac arrest may develop due to heart attack, electric shock, suffocation, choking after severe injury or allergic reactions etc.

As soon as heart stops beating and breathing also stops, the person is considered clinically dead but the vital centres of C.N.S. remain viable for 4-6 minutes more. If during this period CPR is given then the life of the victim may be revived.

Cardio-pulmonary resuscitation can be performed under following steps :

    (a) Clearance of airway.
    (b) Artificial breathing.
    (c) Cardiac massage.

(a) Clearance of Airway

First of all the air passage should be opened and cleaned so as to make a free passage for air. For this purpose wrap a handkerchief or a piece of clean cloth on your first two fingers together and clean victim's mouth taking care that his breathing is not blocked. During cleaning process the mouth of the patient should be turned to a side so that the particles of cleaned material may not fall in the respiratory tract.

(b) Artificial Breathing

Without food a person can survive for 70 days, without water he can survive for 7 days but without air a person cannot survive for more than 3-4 minutes. Therefore whenever breathing is stopped the patient should be immediately given artificial respiration also known as pulmonary resuscitation to save his life.

1. Mouth to Mouth Resuscitation

There are several methods of artificial respiration but mouth to mouth method is considered as effective and easiest method to be used. During this method air is blown from the mouth of first aider into the mouth of the victim who suffers from respiratory failure.

Technique of Mouth to Mouth Respiration

    (i) Place the patient horizontally on his back on a hard flat surface.

(ii) Loosen clothings around his neck and remove any artificial teeth.

(iii) Clear the airway with a handkerchief. During this process mouth of the victim should be turned to a side so as to prevent entry of the particles into the respiratory tract.

(iv) Tilt the head backwards with one hand and support the neck with other hand. This will lift the tongue to its normal position. Thus the airway will be cleared and the patient may start breathing on his own.

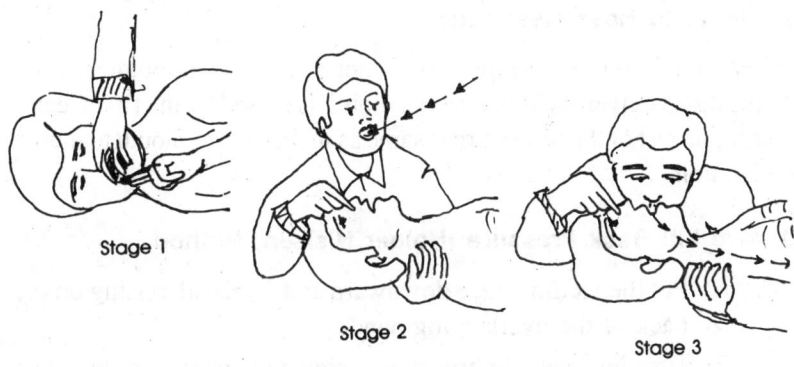

Stage 1

Stage 2

Stage 3

Fig. 4.1 : Mouth to mouth respiration.

(v) If the breathing does not start, pinch the patient's nostrils together, take a deep breath, then seal the patient's mouth tightly with your own mouth and breath out the air forcefully into his lungs. Now move up your head and inhale more fresh air from the atmosphere, again seal patient's mouth with your own mouth and breath out the air forcefully into his lungs. Repeat this process rapidly a number of times so as to saturate the patient's blood with oxygen. Afterwards 12 breathings per minute should be given to an adult patient. Continue this procedure till the patient starts breathing on his own.

Pinching the nose during mouth to mouth respiration is very important because the nose and mouth are connected with each other by an air passage. If the nose is kept open, air would go out through the nose and will not enter into the lungs where it is needed. In the same way if mouth to nose method is used for artificial respiration then victim's mouth must be kept closed if the process is to work.

In certain situations, mouth to mouth respiration cannot be given i.e.

    (i) When the face is damaged;

    (ii) When the jaw is fractured;

    (iii) When lips and mouth have been burned by a poison; or

    (iv) Due to any other reason

then mouth to nose or other manual methods of artificial respiration may be used.

2. Mouth to Nose Respiration

When mouth to mouth respiration is not possible then mouth to nose respiration is given. In this case the mouth is closed by the first aider's palm. The rest of the procedure is same as in the case of mouth to mouth respiration.

3. Arm Lift Back Pressure (Holger Nielsen) Method

    (i) Put the victim's face downward and forehead resting on the back of the overlapping hands.

    (ii) Turn his head slightly to one side and ensure that his jaws are open. This is done to ensure that the air passage is completely open and free; and the particles present in the mouth may not enter into the air passage.

    (iii) Kneel at the victim's head looking towards his feet, placing one knee near the head and the opposite foot by the side of the corresponding side elbow. The position of the knee and the foot may be changed from time to time.

    (iv) Place both hands on his back and spread the palms just in the centre of the shoulders.

    (v) Keep the arms and forearms straight. Lean forward so as to apply even pressure, downward on your hands.

    (vi) Count one-two and lean back. Immediately pull the arms of the patient and lift them up, counting three and keeping your upper limbs straight. Count four-five and then lower the patient's arms back to its original position.

    (vii) Repeat this whole process about 12 times a minute till the respiration of the patient is revived.

(viii) Clean the mouth of the patient from time to time to keep it clean.

This method is not suitable if the patient has severe injuries of chest or arms.

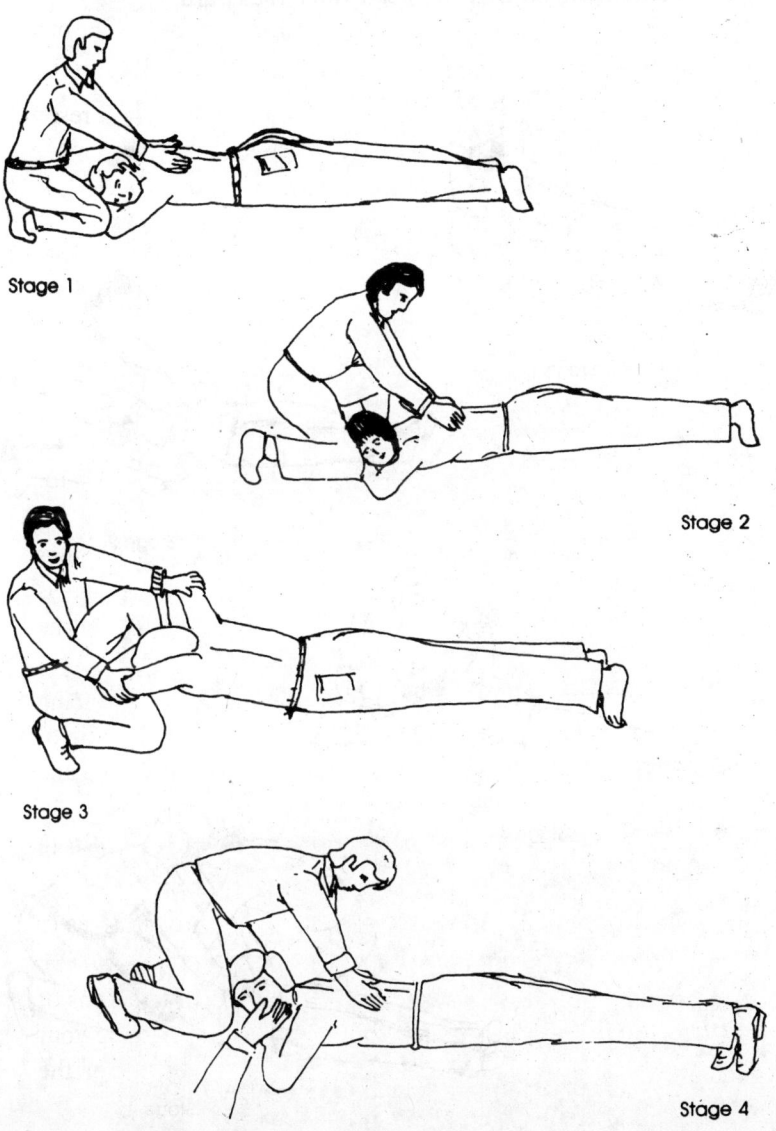

Stage 1

Stage 2

Stage 3

Stage 4

Fig. 4.2 : Artificial respiration. Arm lift back pressure (Holger Nielsen) method.

4. Arm Lift Chest Pressure (Silvester) Method

(i) Put the victim on his back so that the face is upward.

(ii) Raise his shoulders by keeping a folded blanket under the shoulders so that the head falls backward.

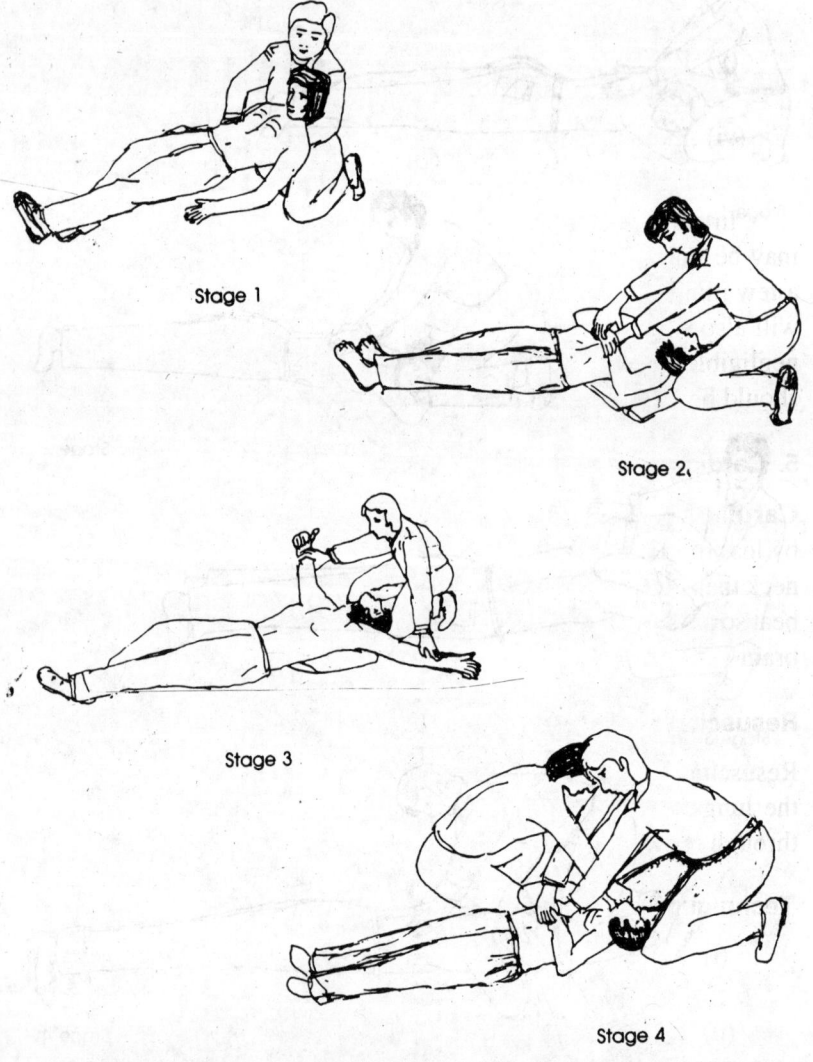

Stage 1

Stage 2

Stage 3

Stage 4

Fig. 4.3 : Artificial respiration. Arm lift chest pressure (Silvester) method.

(iii) Kneel at victim's head. Grasp his forearms near wrist, cross them and press them over the lower part of the chest. The pressure should cause the air to flow out from victim's nose and mouth.

(iv) Immediately pull the arms upwards and outwards over his head with a sweeping movement and place them backward as far as possible for 3 seconds.

(v) Repeat the whole cycle for 12 times a minute and go on repeating till respiration is revived.

(vi) Keep the mouth as clean as possible at all times during respiration.

In certain cases of accidents, even if the breathing has stopped, may be due to any reason, the heart may still continue to beat but for a few minutes only and if respiration is not revived the heart beating will also stop then the chances of survival of the patient will be very negligible. Therefore in such cases cardiopulmonary resuscitation should be immediately started.

5. Cardiopulmonary Resuscitation

Cardiac Massage : If the heart stops beating which can be diagnosed by loss of consciousness, failure to feel the pulse at the wrist or in the neck then cardiac massage should be started at once to revive the heart beat so as to circulate the blood to various organs of the body including brain.

Resuscitation

Resuscitation is the process of maintaining the exchange of gases in the lungs through artificial respiration and revival of heart activity through resuscitation method.

Technique of Cardiac Massage

(i) Place the victim horizontally on the ground or on a flat, hard surface with face in the upward position.

(ii) Kneel on the side of the chest of the victim.

(iii) Place the right hand two fingers above the lower end of the sternum.

(iv) Place the left hand over the right hand.

(v) At this place press the breast bone down towards the spine for about 4 cm in an adult. Remember that pressure is applied at exactly the correct position and while applying pressure only the heel of the hand comes in contact with the chest wall.

(vi) After applying pressure for about half second, release the pressure after each compression, completely relax the pressure so that the sternum returns to the normal position. Compression and relaxation time should be equal.

(vii) Repeat the cycle 60-70 times a minute for an adult. It should be a continuous cycle without removing the hands from the position.

If the breathing and heart beating both are absent then you should immediately start artificial breathing and external cardiac massage together in a rhythmic manner. If you are alone performing CPR, then give 15 heart compressions; rush to the head side and give two mouth to mouth breathings, get back to the heart and again give 15 compressions. If two persons are performing CPR, one should do cardiac massage and the other should give mouth to mouth respiration. Here, after every 5 heart compressions, one mouth to mouth breathing should be given to the patient. The cycle is repeated until the breathing

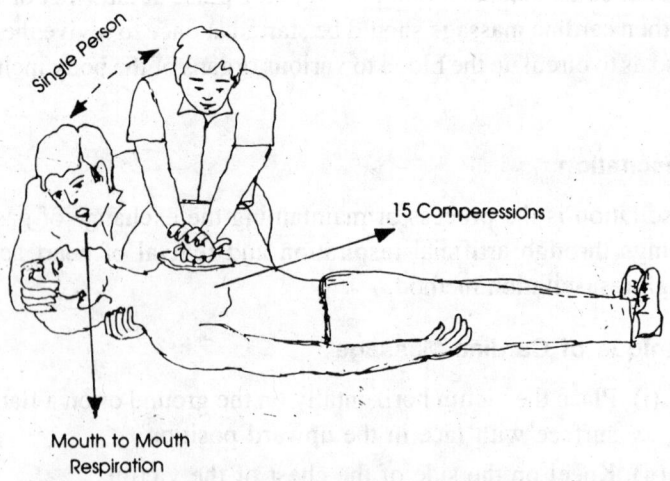

Fig. 4.4 : Cardiopulmonary resuscitation by a single person.

and heart beating comes to normal. If the treatment is effective the following signs will appear :

(i) Colour of the face and skin will become normal.

(ii) Pupil will start contracting.

(iii) Pulsation and heart beating will be felt.

Note :

1. Do not begin thumping the heart or heart massage until it is very necessary or you are sure that the heart has stopped beating. The necessity of cardiac massage will be shown by the signs :

(i) Bluish face.

(ii) Pupil dialated and non-reactive to light.

(iii) Absence of pulsation and heart beating.

2. Wrong and careless pressure applied may cause injury to the ribs and deeper tissues.

3. Even if the patient is breathing but the breathing is not normal, it is wise to start artificial respiration.

4. If heart beat and respiration is not normal start cardiac massage and mouth to mouth respiration simultaneously.

5. If a period of 5 minutes or more has passed from the time of cessation of cardiac functions to the start of CPR then the chances sto revive these functions will be negligible.

5

ENVIRONMENT
AND HEALTH

The term environment includes all the aspects surrounding a man. It includes internal, external, living and non-living aspects.

Internal environment includes all tissues and organs of a body which should work in coordination with each other.

In modern concept the external environment includes not only water, air and soil that form our environment but also include social and economic aspects. Broadly speaking the external environment includes the following components :

(i) **Physical** : These include water, air, food, soil, season, climate, housing, facilities for disposal of excreta and other waste products.

(ii) **Chemical** : These include insecticides, pesticides, fertilizers used in agricultural production and chemicals present in industrial wastes.

(iii) **Biological** : These include plants, animals, rodents, insects and micro-organisms.

(iv) **Social** : These include society, culture, customs, occupation, religion, personal habits, income and standard of living.

The body maintains an equilibrium between the internal and external environment but sometimes the state of equilibrium is disturbed and diseases are caused.

ENVIRONMENTAL SANITATION

For the causation of any diesease three factors i.e. agent, host and environment are necessary. Out of these, agent and host are the known factors but environment is unknown which is a very important link between agent and host to transmit a disease. If environmental factors are controlled they may help in the prevention of diseases. The control of environmental factors in disease causation is known as environmental sanitation which means "the science of safeguarding health". According to WHO the environmental sanitation is defined as "the control of all those factors in man's physical environment which exercise or may exercise a deleterious effect on his physical development, health and survival". The term environmental sanitation is now replaced with environmental health, which is an important component of community health.

ENVIRONMENTAL HEALTH

Environmental pollution is the major reason which causes harmful effects on man's health and leads to so many diseases. The environmental pollution occurs through pollution of water, air and soil; unhygienic disposal of human excreta and refuse; insects and rodents. Poor housing facilities also add to the problem of environmental sanitation.

Rapid population growth and industrial development have led to exploitation of natural resources. Water, air and soil are being polluted. Forests are being finished which has resulted in climatic imbalances, therefore, changes are taking place in seasons as well.

In India, if safe drinking water is provided to everybody, excreta and other waste materials are disposed of in a sanitary manner and air is kept pollution free then a large number of infectious diseases can be prevented. Therefore now a days a great stress is being laid on environmental sanitation.

WATER

Water is essential for life next to air. Without water there would have been no life. Due to this reason in early times man had the tendency to settle near sources of water e.g. near rivers, lakes and springs etc. But now a days where new colonies are developed provision of safe drinking water is made.

Though all efforts are made to provide safe drinking water to the public but still in India more than half of the rural population is not getting safe drinking water. It has been estimated that more than 50 percent of diseases in India can be decreased if safe drinking water alone is provided to the public living in slums and rural areas.

Safe and wholesome water is that water which is free from harmful pathogenic micro-organisms and harmful chemical substances. It is pleasant in taste and does not harm the user even if it is used continuously for prolonged periods.

Uses of Water

Our body contains about two thirds of water of its total weight. Blood contains 79%, brain 80% and bones about 10% of water. Hence water is an integral part of body. It is required to perform the following functions:

(i) It helps in the digestion of food.

(ii) It helps in the secretion of digestive juices.

(iii) It maintains electrolyte balance in the body.

(iv) It helps in the conduction of nerve impulses.

(v) It maintains the fluidity of blood, lymph and all secretions.

(vi) It maintains the body temperature and acts as a distributor of body heat.

(vii) It helps in the excretion of waste products from the body.

Apart from body needs of water, it is required for following purposes :

(a) **Domestic Purposes** : For drinking, cooking, bathing and washing etc.

(b) **Public Purposes** : For cleaning public places, for gardens, swimming pools and for fire fighting etc.

(c) **Industrial Purposes** : All types of industries require water for one purpose or the other. Some industries like iron and steel industries and paper industries require water in huge amounts.

(d) **Agricultural Purposes** : Agriculture is based on water. If there is no water there will be no vegetation.

Water Requirements

The amount of water required per head depends on climatic conditions, standard of living and personal hygienic habits. The water requirement depends on type of industry. Similarly different types of agricultural crops need varying amounts of water. For public use a daily supply of 200 to 400 litres in a standard family is considered reasonable. The requirement increases in summer season.

Sources of Water

The main sources of water are :

1. Rain.
2. Surface water i.e. artificial lakes, rivers, canals, streams, ponds and tanks.
3. Ground water i.e. wells and springs.

1. RAIN

Rain is the primary source of all water sources. When it rains a large amount of rain water sinks into the earth to form ground water. A part of rain water is converted into streams and rivers which ultimately meet in the sea. A part of rain water gets evaporated. This evaporated water forms clouds and comes back to the earth in the form of rain. This cycle known as 'water cycle' goes on.

Rain water is the purest form of water in nature. It is clear, bright, very soft and is comparable to distilled water. It is also free from micro-organisms. But rain water gets contaminated as it passes through the atmosphere and reaches the ground. These impurities are dust, soot, suspended matter, gases and even microorganisms. But all these impurities are not of much importance, since they are not pathogenic like germs of cholera, typhoid fever etc. The first rain which falls on the earth is not pure it may be contaminated with dust, soot, pollen grains, insects and other suspended particles in the air. Rain water collected after sufficient rain is good and useful for cooking, bathing and washing purposes. But it must be collected and stored properly. However rain water has one serious drawback that since it is soft therefore it dissolves lead from lead pipes and may cause lead poisoning. This disadvantage can be overcome if instead of lead pipes other kinds of pipes are used.

2. SURFACE WATER

When rain water reaches on ground or melted snow from the hills begins to flow in the form of streams, rivers and canals or is collected in lakes, ponds or tanks it is called surface water. Rain water and snow are the major sources of surface water and in turn surface water is the most important source of water because in India most of the cities and villages depend on it for their water needs.

(a) Artificial Lakes

These are lakes which are constructed in the upland areas to store water which runs on the sides of hills, slopes and valleys before it forms big streams and rivers. The water may be collected in the form of natural lakes or artificially constructed lakes e.g. in Simla, Madras, Bombay and Darjeeling. The area from which the water is collected in the reservoir or lake is called 'catchment area'. The catchment area should be free from any contamination otherwise the water may get contaminated. Therefore this area should be kept free from grazing of cattles and human habitations.

The upland water collected in this way is safe and good quality water because it is pure rain water which has travelled short distance but even then this water should be purified by filtration and sterilized by chlorination before final storage.

(b) Rivers

Rivers, canals and streams are another major source of water. Many cities like Delhi, Agra, Calcutta and Ahmedabad get their water supply from rivers. The major supply of water to the city beautiful 'Chandigarh' is from a canal 'The Bhakra Mainline Canal'. Most of rivers in India are a continuous and permanent source of water supply. Since rivers travel a long distance passing through the sides of big cities therefore they get contaminated and their water becomes unfit for human consumption. Since rivers are open spaces so people freely use it for defaecation, bathing, washing, and bring their cattle for drinking and bathing purposes.

Dead bodies are burnt on the banks of rivers. Sewage, industrial waste and water from agriculture land is thrown into the rivers. On holy occasions thousands of pilgrims take bath at a time resulting in addition to the pollution of water.

Since water in rivers, canals and streams is running water so it automatically gets purified to certain extent i.e. by the process of dilution, sedimentation, oxidation and by ultraviolet rays present is sunlight. This natural purification of water is not sufficient therefore river, canal or stream water must be purified and sterilized before it is stored for human consumption.

(c) Tanks and Ponds

Tanks and ponds are important sources of water supply in some of villages where there is no other source of water supply and the rain is also scanty. These are artificially made and are used to store rain water. Tank water, like river water is never safe for drinking and domestic purposes because all the filth and garbage of the surrounding areas is washed directly into these tanks and ponds during rainy season. People themselves contaminate the water of tanks and ponds by bathing and washing. They defaecate on the banks of ponds. Animals also drink water and sometimes children swim in these tanks and ponds. So the pond or tank water is the most polluted water therefore must not be used for human consumption unless it is purified.

Tanks and ponds are good sources of water supply in villages if they are protected, maintained and kept pollution free. This can be achieved if following measures are taken :

(i) It should be made by exavating a good soil, loose sandy soil should be avoided.

(ii) Its surroundings should be good and there should be no insanitary or borehole laterine nearby.

(iii) Its edges should be raised so as to prevent the entry of water from nearby areas during rainy season.

(iv) It should be properly fenced so as to prevent the entry of animals etc.

(v) No tree should be planted near the tank. They should be planted at a distance.

(vi) Weeds and algae should be periodically removed.

(vii) Bathing and washing in the tank and pond should be strictly prohibited.

(viii) Jute steeping etc. should not be allowed in the tanks and ponds.

(ix) Water should be drawn out from an elevated platform by a hand pump.

If the above precautions are followed then and only then water from a tank or pond should be used for human consumption that too after purification.

3. GROUND WATER

The part of rain water which sinks into the ground and reaches in subsoil to a varying depths is known as ground water.

The ground water is considered superior to surface water because:

(i) The ground itself acts as an effective filtration medium.

(ii) The chances of contamination are less.

(iii) No treatment for purification is required.

(iv) The supply remains almost constant throughout the year even during summer season.

The disadvantages of ground water are that it is harder than surface water and it requires pumping to take out water from ground. The sources of ground water are wells and springs.

(A) WELLS

Wells are the main source of water supply in most Indian villages and towns. They are artificial holes or pits dug into the earth to reach to the underground water level. The water collected in the pits is taken out manually or mechanically.

Types of Wells

There are four types of wells :

(i) Shallow wells

(ii) Deep wells

(iii) Tube wells

(iv) Artesian wells

(i) Shallow Wells

Shallow wells are those wells where subsoil water i.e. ground water lying between the surface and first impermeable layer is tapped. The shallow wells may be less than 10 ft. deep or sometimes they may be more than 30 to 50 feet deep. Most of the wells in India are of shallow type.

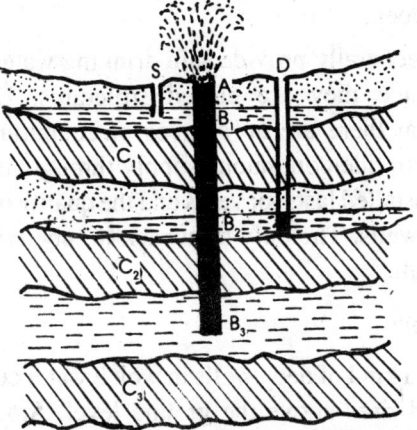

S–Shallow well;   D–Deep well;   A–Artesian well
$B_1B_2B_3$ — Water bearing layer $C_1C_2C_3$ — Impermeable layer

Fig. 5.1 : Different types of wells.

The water of these wells is never safe for drinking purposes unless it is purified. Shallow wells are liable to contamination with sewage and other surface impurities present in the surroundings. They may also get contaminated from dug well latrines, leaking drains, droppings of birds and leaves etc.

(ii) Deep Wells

Deep wells are those wells which penetrate the first impermeable layer and tap the water present under this layer. They may pass through one or more impermeable layers.

Deep well water is safer for drinking purposes as compared to shallow well water on account of efficient filtration because this water travels a greater distance through the earth. They provide permanent supplies than shallow wells. These deep wells can also become a health hazard if they are open, poorly constructed and not protected against contamination.

(iii) Tube Wells

Tube wells are simply shallow wells but here a metallic or plastic pipe is introduced upto 20-25 feet depth to tap the water. The tube is fitted with a screen at the bottom and a mechanical device to draw out water is attached at the top. Like wells, tube wells may also be of two types i.e. shallow and deep.

Tube wells generally provide safe drinking water and free from contamination since they are closed structures. Due precaution must be taken that there are no sources of contamination near the tube well. They provide continuous supply throughout the year. The equipment once installed lasts for years and the quality of water is better than the shallow wells. The only drawback in tube wells is that they are costly to install.

(iv) Artesian Wells

Artesian wells are a kind of deep wells in which water comes out under great pressure and rises above the ground level. Artesian wells are named after Artois province in France where they have been used for a long time. These types of wells are not common in India.

Sanitary Wells

A sanitary well should have the following qualities :

(i) As wells are important source of water so they should be made *pucca*.

(ii) It should be made in a good soil and should be at least 50 ft. away from any possible source of contamination.

(iii) The location of the well should not be very close to the living places and not very far off which may be inconvenient for the user to fetch water from there.

(iv) The site should be at a higher level to prevent entry of surface water into the well.

(v) It should be a deep well i.e. sunk below the first impermeable layer.

(vi) Its walls should be made with bricks and plastered with one inch thick cement from both sides i.e. inside and outside of the well upto 20 feet depth.

(vii) A concrete parapet about 2-3 feet above the ground level should be made. This will prevent the entry of surface water into the well.

(viii) There should be a concrete platform about 1 metre radius around the well. It should have a gentle slope outwards. A *pucca* drain should be provided to carry the spilled water away from the well.

(ix) Roots of trees should not be allowed to sprout from the linings of the wall.

(x) The mouth of the well should be well covered to prevent falling of leaves etc. into the well.

(xi) The water should be drawn with hand pump or with single bucket attached to a rope only.

(xii) People should not be allowed to take bath, wash clothes or clean utensils at the well. However they may be allowed to do so at a short distance away from the well.

(xiii) From time to time the quality of water should be tested in a laboratory to ensure that the water is fit for drinking.

If above mentioned qualities are adhered to and proper cleanliness is maintained around the well then the quality of water obtained from the well will be fairly good and fit for drinking purposes.

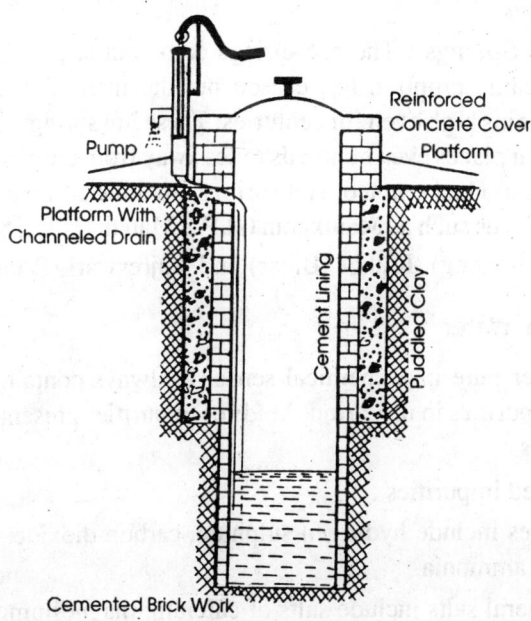

Fig. 5.2 : Protected well.

(B) SPRINGS

Springs are natural outlets of ground water held under pressure by the impermeable layer. They come out at places where the geological conditions are favourable. Their yield of water is usually too small to cater to the needs of a community for water. Their location is not always convenient, so they are not considered as an important source of water.

Types of Springs

There are four types of springs :

(i) **Surface Springs or Shallow or Land Springs :** These are comparable to shallow wells.

(ii) **Deep or Main Springs :** These are comparable to deep wells.

(iii) **Mineral Springs :** The water of these springs contains dissolved mineral salts in high quantities. Therefore, they are used for medicinal or therapeutic uses. Sulphur springs are very common in India. Spring waters containing iron, magnesium and other metal salts are also found at certain places.

(iv) **Hot Springs :** The hot springs come out at places where a volcanic eruption has ceased but the internal temperature remains high even for centuries. These hot springs may come out at places even hundreds miles away from the places where volcano had erupted. Hot springs are quite common in India at places such as Manikaran (H.P.), Manali (H.P.), Sitakoond (Chittagong), Rajkot (Bihar) and Vajreswari (Bombay).

Impurities in Water

Water is never pure in a chemical sense. It always contains certain amount of impurities in it. Various kinds of impurities present in water are as follows :

1. Dissolved impurities :

(a) Gases include hydrogen sulphide, carbon dioxide, nitrogen and ammonia.

(b) Mineral salts include salts of calcium, magnesium, sodium, iron, lead and manganese.

2. Suspended impurities include particles of sand, mud, clay, dust, dead leaves, plants, bacteria, viruses, ova, cysts and insects.

Water Pollution

When natural colour and taste of water is changed and bad smell comes out from water due to any kind of contamination higher than the permitted limits it is known as water pollution. Generally water contains both dissolved and suspended impurities. The dissolved impurities include hydrogen sulphide, carbon dioxide, nitrogen and ammonia and mineral salts. The suspended impurities include sand, mud clay, dry leaves, plants, bacteria etc.

With rapid urbanisation and industrialisation, the pollution of natural water is increasing to an alarming proportion. The disposal of sewage from the townships to the nearby streams and rivers has caused a serious problem of water pollution. Industrial wastes from electroplating, dying, vegetable oil, paper, textile, sugar, jute and iron industries, tanneries and milk plants etc. are also channeled to the streams and rivers. Fertilizers and pesticides from agriculture and from such industries find their way into the streams. All these wastes contain highly toxic chemical substances which are not only harmful for human consumption but agricultural crops, fish and other water animals are also affected by these toxic substances present in industrial wastes. The toxic effects of these chemicals may not be immediately noticed but may produce long term irreversible toxic effects either by consuming water, agriculture products or even fishes.

To prevent pullution of water the Parliament passed an Act in 1974 "Prevention and Control of Water Pollution Act 1974". According to this Act any individual or industry owner found polluting water will be prosecuted.

Water Borne Diseases

Consumption of contaminated water with pathogenic micro-organisms leads to so many diseases known as water borne diseases. These diseases are classified as follows :

(i) **Bacterial Diseases** : Diarrhoea, dysentery, typhoid, paratyphoid and cholera.

(ii) **Viral Diseases** : Poliomyelitis, viral hepatitis.

  (iii) **Protozoal Diseases :** Amoebiasis, giardiasis.
  (iv) **Worm Infestations :** Round worm, thread worm.
  (v) **Other Diseases Due to the Presence of Aquatic Host :** Guinea worm and tape worm.
  (vi) **Diseases Due to Toxic Substances :** Lead, arsenic, cadmium, chromium, copper, mercury etc.

It is estimated that more than 70% population in developing countries specially residing in villages get polluted water. If safe drinking water is provided to them then more than 50 percent diseases can be controlled.

Purification of Water

Water is purified on large scale for supply to a city or a town. It is also purified on small scale for domestic use.

Large Scale Purification of Water

In the purification of water on large scale following methods are used:

  1. Slow sand filtration (biological filtration).
  2. Rapid sand filtration (mechanical filtration).

Slow Sand Filtration

This system was first introduced in England about more than a century ago and still commonly used. Hence it is also known as English system. In slow sand filtration following stages are involved :

  (a) Storage
  (b) Filtration
  (c) Chlorination

(a) Storage.

The raw water from the source, usually a river, canal or a stream is collected in natural or artificial large open reservoirs known as settling tanks. The water is allowed to remain there for 1 to 2 days. During this short period of storage natural purification takes place. About 90 percent suspended impurities settle down by gravity. The organic matter present in the water is oxidised by bacteria with the help of dissolved oxygen present in water. The number of micro-organisms present also decreases considerably. The turbidity due to mud etc. also decreases. At this stage the quality of water improves to a great extent and water becomes much clearer in appearance.

(b) Filtration

Filtration is the second stage in the purification of water and is very important stage because about 99 percent bacteria are removed at this stage. During filtration the clarified water from storage tanks is now admitted to the slow sand filters. The filter beds are water tight rectangular tanks made up of concrete. Usually they are arranged side by side and generally kept open. At least two filtration beds must be constructed so that one must remain in function when the other one is being cleaned. The size of the tanks depends on the requirement of water to be supplied to the community. These beds are generally 2.5 to 4 metres deep.

The filtration bed or sand bed is the most important component because the water is to be filtered through this bed.

They are filled from bottom to upward as follows :

(i) The lowest layer consists of 4 cm size gravel or broken stones.

(ii) Above this layer there is fine gravel. The total thickness of gravel layer is 15-30 cm.

(iii) The third layer above the fine gravel is of coarse sand. The thickness of this layer should be 15 to 30 cm. The gravel layer gives support to the sand layer.

(iv) The fourth layer above the coarse sand layer is of fine sand. The thickness of this layer should be from 60 to 90 cm. As the particles of sand are very small and large in number, they provide large surface area for the water to pass through. Apart from mechanical straining, oxidation, sedimentation and removal of bacteria also takes place.

(v) On the top of these layers there is layer of clarified water from settling tank, about 1.5 to 1.8 metres in height. The inlet of water is controlled by valves fitted at the top of the filter bed. At the bottom of the bed a number of perforated pipes are fitted to collect the filtered water.

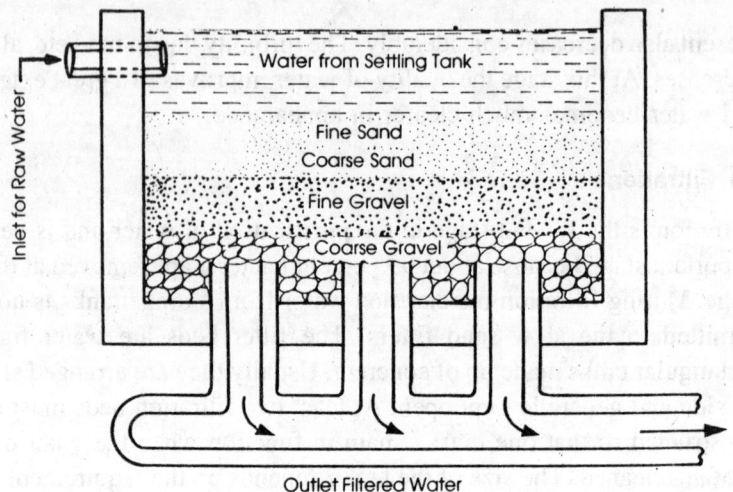

Inlet for Raw Water

Water from Settling Tank

Fine Sand
Coarse Sand
Fine Gravel
Coarse Gravel

Outlet Filtered Water

Fig. 5.3 : Slow sand filter.

No doubt all the components of filter bed specially the sand play a great role in the filtration of water but the vital layer which is formed at the surface of sand plays the greatest role in the purification of water. This is a thin green slimy gelatinous layer which consists of numerous forms of plant and animal life e.g. algae, fungi, protozoa and bacteria. The process of formation of vital layer is known as "ripening" of the filter. This layer is formed within 2-3 days on a new filter bed and when fully formed it is about 2-3 cm in thickness. As the thickness of this vital layer goes on increasing, with the passage of time, the filtration goes on decreasing. After sometime when the thickness increases to a great extent (about 4 feet) and filtration reduces then cleaning of the filter is done. For cleaning, the top sand layer is scraped off. This process of cleaning the filter is repeated periodically. When after repeated cleanings the thickness of sand layer reduces to about 30-40 cm, the plant is closed down and a new bed is prepared. This is usually done after an interval of three years.

The new filter takes about 3 days to work effectively because it takes 2-3 days for the vital layer to form. So the water received during first three days should be allowed to go waste and purified water should be supplied only when bacteriological examination of water shows that efficient filtration is taking place.

Advantages of Slow Sand Filters : Slow sand filters have the following advantages :

(i) They are easy to prepare.

(iii) They are more practicable for filtration of water in developing countries with mininum filtration. They were first used in 1804 in Scotland. Even today they are accepted as standard method of purification of water all over the world.

(iv) They yield 98-99% bacteria free water.

Disadvantages

(i) More land is required for their construction so initial cost is much more than rapid sand filters.

(ii) They require periodical cleaning.

2. Rapid Sand Filtration (Mechanical Filtration)

Rapid sand filters were first introduced in 1885 in U.S.A. Since then they have gained considerable popularity and are still commonly used.

Types of Rapid Sand Filters : There are two types of rapid sand filters:

(i) Gravity type e.g. Paterson's filter.

(ii) Pressure type e.g. Candy's filter.

The Paterson's rapid filter is more commonly used. During rapid filtration 5 steps are involved which are discussed below :

(a) Coagulation

(b) Mixing

(c) Flocculation

(d) Sedimentation

(e) Filtration

(a) **Coagulation :** The water from the setting tanks is led continuously into the plant. Here the water is treated with a chemical coagulant such as alum to remove turbidity and colour. The amount of alum used is 5 to 40 mg per litre, depending upon the amount of turbidity present in the water.

(b) **Mixing :** The alum treated water is then agitated mechanically in a mixing chamber for a few minutes so as to dissolve the alum and the impurities get precipitated.

(c) **Flocculation :** The water is then passed into the flocculation chamber where it is stirred at a slow speed for about half an hour so as to form floccules of aluminium hydroxide.

(d) **Sedimentation :** The coagulated water is then led to the settlement tank where the precipitates are allowed to settle at the bottom of the settlement tank. The water is allowed to remain there for 2 to 6 hours. During this time the precipitates along with suspended matter and bacteria settle at the bottom and the supernatant water now looks very clear in appearance. The flocculated material from the settlement tank is removed from below.

(e) **Filtration :** Filtration is the most important step in the rapid sand filtration process. The clarified water is led to the rapid sand filter which purifies water from 98-99 percent.

In rapid sand filters the medium of filtration is like that of slow sand filtration i.e. sand and gravel. The filter is made up of concrete chamber about 7 feet deep which contains filtering medium i.e. sand supported by gravel. The thickness of filtering medium should be 4 to 5 feet. The filtered water is collected through a network of perforated pipes attached at the bottom of the filter.

Cleaning of the Filters

As the filtration proceeds, after 6-7 days, a layer similar to vital layer in slow sand filters, develops due to collection of floccules which were not sedimented; suspended matter and bacteria. As a result of continuous filtration the filter bed becomes dirty and requires cleaning of filters.

For cleaning the filters washing process known as 'back washing' is done. During this process the inlet and outlet valves are closed. A backflow of purified water from the clean reservoir is made through the bottom of sand bed with simultaneous stirring of the upper layer of sand by means of rotatory metal arms or a blast of compressed air. In this way the deposited layer of floccules and suspended matter will be dislodged and removed with wash water. When the sand looks clear the washing should be stopped. The entire process of washing takes about 15 to 20 minutes and the filters are ready for use again within another 20 minutes. This is an advantage over slow sand filtration where the entire bed needs reconstruction.

Advantages

(i) Very little space is required.

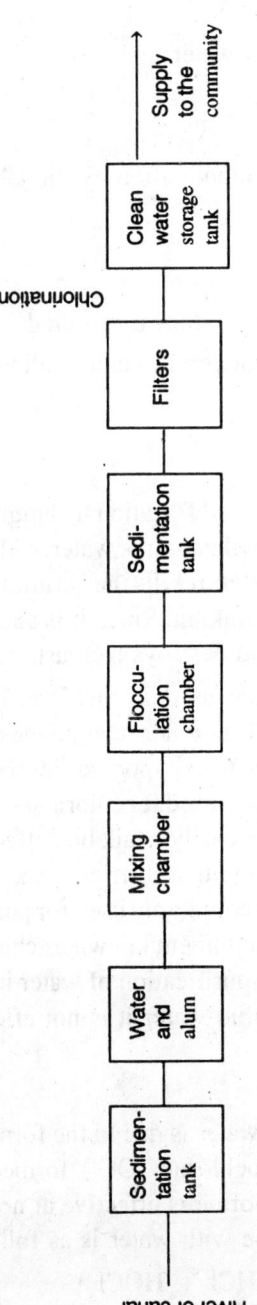

Fig 5.4 : Flow diagram of rapid sand filtration plant.

  (ii) Initial cost is less.

 (iii) They are suitable for turbid water.

 (iv) Water is filtered rapidly.

  (v) Cleaning the filter is easy.

 (vi) There are no chances of contamination by the labourers.

Disadvantages

  (i) Running costs are high.

 (ii) A chemical coagulant such as alum is required.

(iii) Results of purification are not good so chlorination of water is required.

(c) Chlorination

Whether slow sand filtration or rapid sand filtration technique is used chlorination of water is required for sterilization of water. Chlorination is the last step in the purification of water. It kills the harmful bacteria, if any and makes the water safe for drinking. Since it is an oxidising agent so it oxidises organic matter and destroys bad taste and smell.

For chlorination chlorine may be used in the form of gas or solution or as bleaching powder. The other compounds include chloramine and perchlorone or high test hypochlorite (HTH) but chlorine is the best choice. Chlorine gas is used for chlorination of large quantities of water because it is cheap, easily available, effective and quick in action but has the disadvantage that it irritates the eyes and poisonous in action. But even then it is commonly used for purification of water. It is applied with a special equipment known as chlorination equipment. When chlorine is used for purification of water it must be ensured that the water is clear, in turbid water it is not effective.

Action of Chlorine

The chemical action of chlorine with water is due to the formation of hypochlorous acid (HOCl) and hypochlorite (OCl) formed in the reaction. The germicidal action of chlorine is effective at neutral pH i.e. around 7. The reaction of chlorine with water is as follows :

$$H_2O + Cl_2 \longrightarrow HCl + HOCl$$
(Hypochlorous acid)

$$HOCl \longrightarrow H + OCl$$
(Hypochlorite)

Before chlorination the amount of chlorine to be used 'chlorine demand' for disinfecting the water is determined. The chlorine demand of water can be determined in the laboratory. For this purpose a known amount of chlorine is added to water, after half an hour the undissolved amount is calculated. The difference between the two values gives the amount of chlorine dissolved in water. When the process of disinfection is complete and if more chlorine is added the free chlorine will start appearing in water. The point where free chlorine appears in water is called 'break point'.

Free Residual Chlorine

After the addition of chlorine, at least one hour time is allowed for the chlorine to produce its action. This time period is called 'contact period'. During this period chlorine kills the bacteria and oxidises the organic matter.

It is the general practice during chlorination of water that from safety point of view a little excess amount of chlorine is added than actually required. This small excess of chlorine is called 'free residual chlorine'. The usual amount of free residual chlorine added is 0.5 mg per litre at the end of one hour chlorination. If more chlorine is added it gives its own taste and smell to water therefore excess amount of chlorine is not acceptable. Hence the total amount of chlorine required for disinfection of water is chlorine demand plus 0.5 mg/litre free residual chlorine.

Small Scale Purification of Water

Water on small scale such as for domestic purposes can be purified as follows :

 (i) Boiling
 (ii) Distillation
 (iii) Filtration through muslin cloth.
 (iv) Three pitcher system.
 (v) Chemicals.
 (vi) Domestic filters e.g. Berkefeld filter and Pasteur's Chamberland filter.

(i) Boiling

Boiling is the oldest and satisfactory method of purification of water on small scale. Boiling for 5 to 10 minutes kills bacteria, spores, cysts and ova of intestinal parasites. It also removes hardness of water and soft water is produced. Boiling is an excellent method of purification of water provided boiling is done in a neat and clean vessel and after boiling it is stored in clean covered container. Preferably water should be boiled in the same container in which it is to be stored. Only that much amount of water should be boiled which can be used within a few hours.

(ii) Distillation

Distillation is also a good method of purification of water. During this method all kinds of dissolved impurities can be removed even the volatile one as well. For this purpose first and last portion of the distillate must be rejected because these portions may contain the volatile ingredients which may again contaminate the distilled water. Distillation is not possible for the purification of water to be used for routine household purposes.

(iii) Filtration through Muslin Cloth

Muslin cloth acts as a coarse filter which can remove the suspended materials. So water filtered through muslin is not fit for drinking purposes though it can be used for other household purposes like bathing, washing the clothes etc.

(iv) Three Pitcher System

This is very old system of purification of water. In this system three pitchers are used which are kept one above the other on a wooden stand. The top picher contains sand, second charcoal and sand; and the lowest collects the purified water. The raw water is filled in the first pitcher from where it percolates through a hole into the 2nd pitcher. From here the water further percolates through the hole to the third pitcher.

(v) Chemicals

Various types of chemical agents used for disinfection of water are discussed as follows :

(a) **Bleaching Powder (Chlorinated Lime) :** Chemically it is $CaOCl_2$. A fresh sample of bleaching powder contains 33% of available chlorine but on storage it looses chlorine content. Therefore bleaching powder is stored in dry, air-tight containers and at cool and dark places. Roughly speaking 2.5 gm of a good quality of bleaching powder could be required to disinfect 1000 litres of water. Bleaching powder will not directly purify the turbid and polluted water. Therefore such water should first be treated with preliminary filtration and then subjected to chlorination.

(b) **Chlorine tablets :** These tablets are good for disinfecting small quantities of water. They are available in different strengths for disinfecting various quantities of water. One tablet of 500 mg is sufficient for disinfecting 20 litres of water. These are available in the market under various trade names e.g. halazone tablets manufactured by the Boots company.

(c) **Quick Lime (Calcium Oxide) :** Some people prefer to use dry slaked lime than ordinary lime. About 360 mg of slaked lime will disinfect 4.5 litres of water. It is cheap, easily available and quite effective. Therefore it is recommended for disinfecting wells and tanks in cholera outbreak. Disadvantage of quick lime is that large doses of it are required for disinfection of water i.e. 20 times than that of bleaching powder.

(d) **High Test Hypochlorite (HTH) :** It is a calcium compound and contains about 65 to 75 percent of available chlorine. This is much stable compound and 1 gm of HTH is needed for one cubic metre of water.

(e) **Alum :** Alum is not a germicidal. It is used to purify muddy water and to remove turbidity. 60 to 240 mg of alum can purity 4-5 litres of water. Calcium carbonate which is present in all kinds of water also gets precipitated as calcium sulphate and aluminium hydrate. The suspended impurites as well as bacteria also get precipitated which are removed after filtration and a clear purified water is obtained.

(f) **Potassium Permanganate :** It is a strong oxidising agent and can kill cholera vibrios but it does not destroy other disease producing organisms.It is used for disinfecting wells. Its dose is 0.5 parts per million (0.5 ppm). It is not suitable for disinfecting large volume of water. Its disadvantages are that it alters the taste, smell and colour of water thus treated. Moreover this method is not considered dependable therefore no longer used for disinfecting the water.

(g) **Bromine and Iodine :** They are not routine disinfectants. They can be used only in emergencies. The dose of bromine is 3.5 mg per litre of water and iodine 2 ppm of water. They can disinfect water within half an hour.

(vi) Domestic Filters

Water for drinking purposes can be purified by means of domestic filters which are discussed below :

(a) **Berkefeld Filters :** These are cylindrical filters known as 'filter candles' or 'ceramic candles'. They are made up of unglazed porcelain or kieselguhr and are available in various porosity grades. When water is purified through these candles the pores get clogged which need cleaning from time to time at least once a week by scrubbing with a hard brush and passing the water under pressure from inside to outside direction which will remove the entangled particles from the interstices.

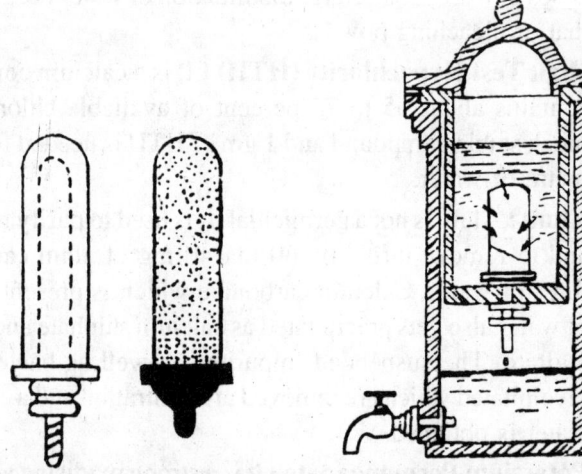

Fig. 5.5 A : Berkefeld filter.   **Fig. 5.5 B :** Berkefeld filtration.

(b) **Pasteur's Chamberland Filter :** It is made up of unglazed porcelain tubes which can be screwed on to a water tap. They work only under pressure and muddy water cannot be filtered through it because the pores will be immediately blocked. Therefore such water must be cleaned to remove mud. For cleaning the filters they are scrubbed from outside with a hard brush and water is made to pass under pressure from inside to outside. They are quick and reliable as they make the water free from all kinds of impurities including bacteria.

Disinfection of Wells

Wells are the common sources of water supply in villages so they should be disinfected regularly to keep the water fit for drinking and domestic purposes. Previously potassium permanganate was used for disinfecting wells but now instead of potassium permanganate, bleaching powder is used for this purpose because it is cheap and quite effective disinfectant.

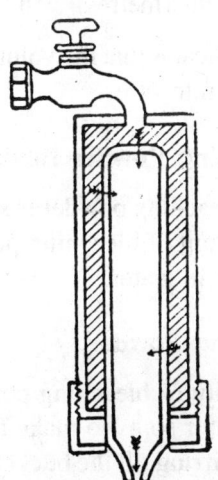

Fig. 56 : Pasteur's Chamberland filter.

For disinfecting the well following steps are involved :

    (i) Measurement of well for its depth.

    (ii) Amount of water in the well.

    (iii) Amount of bleaching powder required.

      (iv) Mixing of bleaching powder.

      (v) Addition of bleaching powder solution in the well.

      (vi) Ortho-toludine test.

(i) Measurement of Well

First of all, the diameter of the well is measured and then its depth is measured in metres by a rope tied with some weight. The rope is lowered in the well till it touches the bottom of the well. Then the rope is taken out and length of the wet portion of the rope is measured which gives height of the water column.

(ii) Amount of Water Present in the Well

In the next step amount of water present in the well is calculated from the following formula :

$$V = \pi\, r^2 h \times 1000 \text{ litres}$$

where V = volume of water π = 22/7

               r = radius (metres) h = height (metres)

      The figure 1000 indicates that the volume is multiplied with 1000 to convert cubic metres into litres.

(iii) Amount of Bleaching Powder Required

10 gm of good quality bleaching powder is sufficient to disinfect 1500 litres of water. This amount of bleaching powder can vary according to the impurities present in water.

(iv) Mixing of Bleaching Powder

Take the required quantity of bleaching powder in a bucket. To this add small amount of water so as to make a paste. Then add more of water with continuous stirring till the bucket is 3/4 full. Allow to stand the contents of the bucket for 5 to 10 minutes so as to settle the lime. Transfer the supernatant clear liquid (chlorine solution) into another bucket and discard the lime sediment (the lime should not be poured into the well as it increases the hardness of well water).

(v) Addition of Bleaching Powder Solution in the Well

Lower the bucket containing chlorine solution into the well and agitate the water by lowering and drawing up the bucket several times and at the same time going round the well so as to mix the chlorine solution thoroughly with the well water.

Allow the chlorine solution to remain in contact with well water for at least one hour (contact period) and during this period no water should be withdrawn from the well. This will allow the chlorine water to kill the pathogenic micro-organisms.

(vi) Ortho-Toludine Test

After one hour (contact period) ortho-toludine test is performed to know whether water has been properly chlorinated or not i.e. free residual chlorine is tested. If it is less than 0.5 mg per litre (0.5 ppm) then additional quantities of bleaching powder will have to be added.

For performing this test analytical grade ortho-toludine dissolved in 10 percent solution of hydrochloric acid is selected. A sample of chlorinated water is taken in a test tube and 2-3 drops of orthotoludine are added to it. The appearance of yellow colour will indicate that sufficient chlorination has been done but appearance of red colour will indicate that excess chlorination has been done.

In villages no routine ortho-toludine test is performed, usually the wells are disinfected with bleaching powder solution late in the evening and water is drawn only in the next morning. This provides sufficient contact period. During cholera epidemics all wells must be disinfected with bleaching powder solution daily.

Hardness of Water

Some of the waters produce lather easily with soap whereas others produce lather with difficulty. A water which produces lather with difficulty is known as hard water and which produces lather readily with soap is known as soft water. In short, hardness of water is defined as soap destroying power of water. Hardness of water is due to the presence of soluble salts i.e. bicarbonates, chlorides and sulphates of calcium and magnesium. Since all these are soluble salts so they remain dissolved in water and are not removed by filtration.

Disadvantages of Hardness of Water

(i) There is wastage of soap and detergents.

(ii) It is unsuitable for cooking certain vegetables, dal and meat. They take very long time to cook in hard water.

(iii) With hard water clothes are not cleaned properly and they do not have a long life.

(iv) Temporary hard water on boiling leads to deposit of a layer of calcium carbonate on inside walls of boilers and kettles which is known as scaling or furring of boilers. This layer interferes with smooth action of boilers resulting in loss of their efficiency. Sometimes scaling of boilers may lead to bursting of boilers resulting in serious accidents and deaths.

(v) It is harmful for industrial purposes and also shortens the life of pipes and fixtures in the industries.

(vi) It is harmful to the health as in certain cases it may lead to diarrhoea and other digestive disorders.

Types of Hardness of Water

Hardness of water is of two types :

    (a) Temporary hardness.

    (b) Permanent hardness.

(a) Temporary Hardness

Temporary hardness is due to the presence of bicarbonates of calcium and magnesium.

(i) It can be removed by boiling. On boiling the carbon dioxide is expelled out of water and precipitates of calcium carbonate and magnesium carbonate are deposited at the bottom.

$$Ca(HCO_3)_2 \xrightarrow{\text{Boiling}} CaCO_3 + H_2O + CO_2$$

$$Mg(HCO_3)_2 \xrightarrow{\text{Boiling}} MgCO_3 + H_2O + CO_2$$

Boiling is an expensive method of removing hardness of water on a large scale.

(ii) Temporary hardness can also be removed by adding lime or calcium hydroxide (Clark's process) to water. Lime absorbs carbon dioxide and precipitates of calcium carbonate are formed which settle at the bottom and separated by filtration.

$$Ca(HCO_3)_2 + Ca(OH)_2 \longrightarrow 2CaCO_3 + 2H_2O$$

(b) Permanent Hardness

Permanent hardness is due to the presence of chlorides and sulphates of calcium and magnesium. It is not removed by boiling. However it can be removed by following methods :

(i) When sodium carbonate or soda ash is added to water, it removes both temporary and permanent hardness of water. The sulphate of calcium and magnesium is converted into sodium sulphate.

$$CaSO_4 + Na_2CO_3 \longrightarrow Na_2SO_4 + CaCO_3$$

(ii) **Base Exchange or Permutit Process :** This process is used for removal of hardness of water on large scale. Sodium permutit is a loose compound of sodium, aluminium and silica. When hard water is passed through it the calcium and magnesium ions are exchanged with sodium ions thus hardness is removed. Therefore this process is also called "base exchange process". With continuous use the sodium ions in the permutit get exhausted and become unfit for further removal of hardness of water. Therefore at this stage it is regenerated by adding strong solution of sodium chloride whereby calcium and magnesium is displaced by sodium and it again becomes sodium permutit fit to remove the hardness of water.

Air

Air is the most important component of man's environment as well as all living organisms. A man can live for a number of days without food and water but without air we cannot survive beyond a few minutes i.e. 3-4 minutes. Air is vital to maintain life and serves to ensure constant supply of oxygen to the body through the process of respiration. Apart from supplying the life-giving oxygen, air performs many other functions in the body i.e. it carries sound and smell and helps in regulating the body temperature. The air may contain disease producing micro-organisms, dust, smoke and chemicals which may be harmful to the body and may lead to different kinds of diseases.

Pure air is necessary for healthy living. Fresh air acts like a tonic. It stimulates digestion, improves metabolism, strengthens the nervous system and increases the body resistance against diseases. When all these body systems are improved by fresh air definitely a person will feel healthy and cheerful. So the air we breathe in must be pure.

Composition of Air

Air is a mechanical mixture of gases and not a chemical compound. The composition of air may vary from place to place but normally the pure air has the following composition :

Oxygen	20.95%
Nitrogen	79.00%
Carbon dioxide	0.03 to 0.04%

The remaining amount is made up of some gases like argon, neon, krypton, xenon and helium which occur in traces. Along with these, air also contains water vapours and suspended impurities like dust, soot, bacteria, spores and vegetable debris etc.

The composition of fresh air generally remains constant due to certain factors that

(a) Movement of air dilutes and takes away the impurities.

(b) The atmospheric temperature and ultraviolet rays present in sunlight oxidises the organic matter and kill the bacteria.

(c) Rain removes the suspended and gaseous impurities thus helps in cleaning the atmosphere

(d) Green plants play a great role in the purification of air due to their chlorophyll content. They take up carbon dioxide from the atmosphere and give off oxygen. This process is reversed during night time. The exchange of oxygen and carbon dioxide by the plants always goes on thus the atmosphere remains clean.

The outdoor and indoor composition of air always differs because the outdoor air is the fresh air whereas indoor air is always affected by the occupants and their activities. A crowded room may be more suffocating due to consumption of oxygen and release of carbon dioxide by all the occupants. Moreover body smells are added to the air and there is an increase in temperature and humidity due to breathing.

Air Pollution

The term air pollution is applied when there is an excessive concentration of foreign matter in the air which is harmful to health. Now a days it is a major problem affecting the atmosphere and health of the public. Increasing urbanisation and industrialisation are the main causes of air pollution. The other major sources of air pollution are:

(i) Process of respiration in men and animals where carbon dioxide is released to atmosphere specially in rooms occupied by a number of persons.

(ii) Industries are a big source of air pollution specially chemical, fertilizer and metallurgical industries. Brick kilns are other sources of air pollution.

(iii) Burning of coal, oil or agriculture waste produces gases like sulphur dioxide, carbon dioxide and smoke which lead to air pollution.

(iv) With increased industrialisation and urbanisation the number of vehicles has tremendously increased specially in urban areas which is one of the major causes of air pollution. Air pollution from the vehicles is very dangerous because the vehicles move from place to place causing pollution everywhere and giving you trouble at home, in the office, in the shoping centre or on the road.

The vehicles like buses, trucks, tractors and railway engines etc. which run on diesel emit more smoke and looks more obnoxious but the vehicles like cars and two/three wheelers which run on petrol are more dangerous since these vehicles come in close proximity with the public, even in houses and streets. The smoke emitted by petrol vehicles contains carbon monoxide — a poisonous gas. When the engines of vehicles are not properly adjusted or tuned they cause even more pollution.

(v) Decomposition of animal and vegetable matters lead to air pollution. After decomposition they emit very offensive and poisonous gases in which bacteria, moulds and fungi grow very rapidly.

(vi) Natural sources like dust, pollens, fungi and bacteria also cause air pollution. Pathogenic micro-organisms or related diseases are present in the vicinity of patients only and not in the atmosphere.

(vii) Insecticides and pesticides sprayed on plants cause air pollution.

(viii) Nuclear energy programmes also pollute the air.

Although more than 100 pollutants have been identified but smoke, suspended particles, gases like carbon monoxide, sulphur dioxide, hydrogen sulphide, oxides of nitrogen, chlorides, fluorides and cancer producing substances are the major pollutants of air.

Effects of Pollution of Air

(i) Mortality and morbidity rates are increased.

(ii) It affects respiratory functions.

(iii) It leads to destruction of plant and animal life. The production of crops is greatly affected.

(iv) It leads to corrosion of metals.

(v) Polluted air causes great damage to the buildings e.g. the Taj is affected by fumes of oil refinery.

(vi) Sometimes visibility is also decreased.

Air Borne Diseases

As a result of air pollution the commonest disease is chronic bronchitis. It is associated with headache, giddiness, depression, chest pain, cough, fever off and on and generalised weakness. If the air pollution is intense, immediate death may take place due to suffocation. It had taken place in Bhopal gas tragedy in which thousands of people died in a very short time and a large number of others were seriously affected.

The other delayed air borne diseases are tuberculosis, diphtheria, smallpox, chicken pox, measles, whooping cough, pneumococcal pneumonia, common cold, conjunctivitis, dermatitis etc. Dust and industrial pollutants lead to tuberculosis, silicosis and lead poisoning etc.

Prevention and Control of Air Pollution

Following measures may help to check air pollution :

(i) Public should be educated through health education about the harmful effects of air pollution.

(ii) Proper ventilators should be provided in crowded rooms.

(iii) Burning of coal and other agricultural wastes like rice husk as fuel must be stopped and it should be replaced by natural gas or electricity.

(iv) Burning of agricultural wastes in the fields should be stopped.

(v) Felling and cutting of trees should be stopped rather they should be planted in large numbers and vegetation should be grown between industrial and residential areas. The open areas where vegetation is grown for the purification of air are known as green belts.

(vi) Smoking at public places must be prohibited.

(vii) Emission of smoke, harmful and toxic substances in the industries must be checked by enforcing legal measures.

(viii) Motor vehicle act and rules should be strictly enforced and the vehicles emitting higher degree of pollutants should be heavily fined or empounded.

Air pollution is an international problem which is drawing the attention of various scientists and governments of respective countries. In India, various agencies have been assigned to overcome this problem. Pollution control boards have been established to check water, air and other kinds of pollutions.

Noise

A sound becomes noise when it causes disturbances or annoyance to the hearer. The wrong sound in wrong place and at wrong time is also called noise. The sensitivity to noise varies from person to person. A sound may disturb a person but may be agreeable to the other. More pollution is continuously increasing due to development of industry, heavy machinery, technology and modern modes of transportation. Sometimes children also cause loud noise.

Noise is measured in units of decibel (dB), the word Bel is in the memory of Alexander Graham Bell. One decibel is the smallest amplitude which can be heard by the human ear. Animals can distinguish some sounds better than human beings. The approximate sound and noise level values of some operational activities are given below :

Whispering	20 decibels
Quiet library	40 decibels
Normal conversation	60 decibels
Vehicular noise	70-80 decibels
Printing press	80 decibels
Motor car horn	100-120 decibels
Train passing a station	110 decibels
Jet aeroplanes	140 decibels

The recommended maximum noise level is 85 decibels. A noise at 100-120 dB is uncomfortable and at 130-140 dB is painful to ears. Exposure to noise above 160 decibels results in rupture of tympanic membrane and permanent deafness. This may happen due of exposure to sudden noise of an explosive nature.

In India activities like marriages, ceremonies, festivals, religious and political activities are not held without the use of loud –speakers and address systems which cause noise pollution. The use of loud-speakers at the religious places daily in the early morning and evening hours is also a great source of noise pollution. The activities like Jagrans, Ramlilas and marriage ceremonies which are carried out at night time cause noise pollution. The worst affected from these loud-speakers are the students preparing for their examinations, sick and old persons.

Effects of Noise

(i) Loud noise may cause direct injury to the auditory organs resulting in deafness.

(ii) Prolonged exposure to any noise of 80 dB or more is likely to be harmful and may produce fatigue, headache, tinnitus (whistling, ringing or buzzing sound in the ears) vertigo and deafness.

(iii) It leads of annoyance and irritability.

(iv) It interferes with speech.

(v) It leads to inability to concentrate.

(vi) Sleep is disturbed.

(vii) Habit of loud speaking develops.

(viii) It leads to certain accidents in industries.

(ix) Certain physiological changes such as increase in blood pressure, heart rate, sweat, nausea, giddiness and visual disturbances may occur.

Prevention and Control of Noise

(i) **Control the Source of Noise :** The machines producing noise should be segregated and enclosed in a sound proof room. The parts of the machine which produce unwanted sound should be properly oiled, greased, repaired or replaced.

(ii) Sound absorbers should be installed in the industries.

(iii) Workers working in the factories producing more than 100 dB noise must be provided with ear plugs etc. Periodic examination of workers exposed to noise must be carried out.

(iv) 'No horn' or 'silent' zones near hospitals, schools etc. should be demarcated and offenders should be fined.

(v) The use of loud-speakers and address systems should be totally banned from 9 p.m. to 6 a.m.

(vi) Heavy vehicular traffic in residential areas should not be allowed.

(vii) Use of pressure horns should be banned.

(viii) Coolers and other electrical appliances should be noiseless.

(ix) T.V., radio etc. should be played at slow volume which is tolerable to everybody in the house and neighbourhood.

(x) Noise pollution by the vehicles should be checked by suitable adjustments and by fitting noise absorbing devices.

(xi) Automobile workshops should be away from the residential areas.

(xii) Green vegetation and plants should be grown. They help to reduce noise by 8 to 10 decibels.

(xiii) Legal measures should be enforced to check noise pollution.

(xiv) Public should be educated about the hazzards of noise and measures to reduce it as far as they can. Their active co-operation is also essential in controlling the noise pollution.

Now a days a number of very sophisticated instruments are available which not only check the noise level but they also measure the loudness, frequency and duration of noise. Such instruments are very useful in factories and other places where noise is a problem.

Lighting

Good lighting of places of work, streets and roads is necessary for proper visibility. Lighting should neither be strong nor dim. Bad lighting may lead to eye strain, headache, irritability, loss of temper and accidents. In industries inadequate lighting is uneconomical as the output tends to decrease and the accident rate might increase. Strong or bright lighting may produce glare which is dangerous to the eyes and decreases critical vision. The source of light should emit uniform light that means it should not flicker. The distribution of light must be uniform over the whole area of work. There should be no shadows in the field of work as it may interfere with vision. No worker should be allowed to gaze directly at a bright light and every effort should be made that glazing light does not enter the eye. As far as possible fluorescent lighting should be provided as it is economical because less electricity is consumed by them, avoids shadows and provides cool and efficient lighting therefore helps in increasing the efficiency of workers.

Lighting may be natural or artificial. Natural lighting is derived from the sunlight. The buildings and rooms usually get the reflected light from various objects or reflected light from the sky. Intensity of natural lighting depends on the time of day, season and weather. Wherever possible natural lighting should be used because it is economical and has beneficial effects on health as the sun rays contain light rays, heat rays and ultraviolet rays. Moreover it does not cause any pollution. In planning the natural system of lighting the following points must be taken into consideration :

   (i) The objects which obstruct the light should be removed partly or completely.

  (ii) Proper windows regarding their location, number, size and shape should be provided.

 (iii) Too many screens and curtains obstruct the natural light.

 (iv) All glazings and window panes should be kept clean.

  (v) Rooms should be regularly white-washed rather than colour washed because white washing provides better reflection of light.

We cannot depend upon natural lighting all the time i.e. during nights and cloudy days we will have to use some artificial lighting system. Common sources of artificial lighting include candles, kerosene lamps, gas lighting and electric lighting. Out of all these systems electric lighting is more commonly used now a days. Electric lighting does not involve combustion and therefore no oxygen is taken and no waste substances are produced. Candles are used for lighting in emergencies only as they are harmful because their flame is naked and sooty and they are costly. Kerosene lamps are also not very favoured for lighting. Various types of vapour lamps are being used. The neon filled sodium discharge lamp gives out monochromatic yellow light which is quite suitable for highways. Generally tube-lights are more commonly used these days because they consume less electricity hence economical, provide cool and efficient lighting. Use of direct lighting as in the case of table lamps projecting towards working area should be avoided as it may cause eye strain. It should be used only when very fine work is to be done. Indirect light is good for illumination. The light is directed towards ceiling or upper parts of the wall and from there the light is reflected to the working area.

Intensity of artificial light is measured in terms of foot candles. A foot candle is the intensity of light received at a point which is placed at a distance of one foot from the source of light of a standard candle power. A standard candle weighs 75.6 gms and burns 7.2 gms of wax per hour. The electric unit 'watt' is equivalent to 0.88 candle power. A minimum of six foot candles illumination is required for clear visibility. For continuous reading it should be 10 to 15 food candles. The intensity of day light is not measured in terms of foot candles but in units called 'Daylight Factor' (D.F.). This is measured by a special instrument known as daylight factor meter. For clear visibility at least one percent daylight factor should be present in rooms.

Solid Waste Disposal and Control

Common terms used in the disposal and control of solid wastes are as follows :

(i) **Refuse :** Discarded waste matter is called refuse in cities and litter in villages. Solid waste material is also called refuse.

(ii) **Scavanging :** Collection and disposal of refuse which is not carried by the sewers but done by manual labour is called scavanging.

(iii) **Conservancy System :** The collection and disposal of human excreta by manual labour is known as conservancy system.

(iv) **Water Carriage System :** The removal of sewage through sewers and drains is called water carriage system.

(v) **Wastes :** Unwanted solid and liquid material from household, streets, commercial establishments and industries is called waste. Unwanted material which is of no use is to be discarded and this discarded material is called refuse. The refuse or solid waste is the discarded material from houses, streets, commercial, industrial and agricultural activities. The composition of refuse depends upon the source of refuse. The refuse from houses generally contains ash, paper, metal, wood, glass, rags, dust, peelings of fruits and vegetables and left over food etc. Similarly refuse from vegetable and fruit markets contains rotten vegetables and fruits. This type of refuse from rotton vegetables, fruits, waste food is called garbage. Since garbage contains organic matter which gets fermented and decomposed within short time specially in summer and rainy season therefore it must be disposed of as early as possible.

The industrial wastes vary from industry to industry. Usually it contains burnt fuel; metal, wood or glass pieces, paper, dust, chemicals and liquid wastes which are harmful sometimes.

So solid wastes are those substances which are of no use and are thrown outside the houses, shops, streets, roads, industries and agricultural fields etc. Though these waste materials are of no direct use but now a days all waste products are reprocessed to convert them to some useful products again. So now a days a number of men, women, young boys and girls are seen busy in sorting various types of materials from these wastes. They pick up all types of wastes like paper, cardboard, metal, plastic and glass containers; plastic chappals, carry bags, rags, metal pieces etc. After sorting out the items they sell them to the junk dealers who in turn sell them to the industries for reprocessing.

The accumulation of refuse is a health hazard because when it decomposes and ferments it attracts flies, insects, rodents, birds, dogs, pigs and other stray animals who scatter the refuse and increase nuisance. Pathogenic micro-organisms which may be present in refuse find their entry into human body through food contaminated by flies, insects and dust resulting in development of diseases. Water, air and soil may also get polluted. Heaps of refuse present an unsightly appearance and abnoxious odour and causes public nuisance. Therefore refuse should be collected, transported and disposed of in a sanitary manner, as quickly as possible.

Storage and Collection of Refuse

Household refuse should the stored in sanitary dust bins made of tough material and covered by lid. It should be placed out side the house. Street and road side refuse should also be stored in large size public bins by conservancy staff. The refuse from dust bins of nearby houses should also be collected in the public bins.

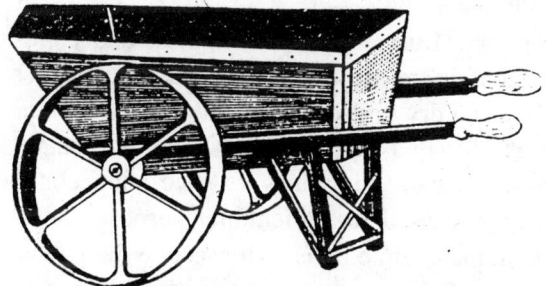

Fig. 5.7 : Wheel barrow or street refuse cart.

For this purpose wheel barrow or street refuse cart can be used. In India since the public is not health conscious, even in urban areas people throw the refuse directly outside the house or the dust bins are emptied on the road side. Even if the public bins are provided they may be far away from houses or they are not emptied for a number of days compelling the users to throw the refuse around or near the bins which is also a nuisance. The refuse from the public bins is carried to distant places for disposal in open vehicles on the main roads which causes a lot of air pollution. The refuse must be carried in covered vehicles to places of disposal and not in open vehicles. Now a days trucks fitted with mechanical devices for tilting the public dust bins directly into the truck for quick and speedy removal of refuse are used in big cities.

In advance countries now a days instead of conventional dust bins paper sacks or polythene sacks are used. Household refuse is stored in the sack and the sack itself is removed with its contents by the conservancy staff for disposal/destruction at a far off place from the habitation and a new sack is kept in its place. This method of refuse collection is becoming very popular in India and is being used specially in hospitals.

Disposal of refuse depends on the circumstances prevailing in the area e.g. availability of land, distance from the collection point, number of persons and vehicles available. The refuse after collection must be disposed of in such a way that it does not create any nuisance. Following methods are used for disposal of refuse :

    (i) Dumping

    (ii) Controlled tipping

    (iii) Burial

    (iv) Compositing

    (v) Burning

  (i) **Dumping :** Dumping is the simplest and easiest method of disposal of dry refuse. Low lying areas away from habitation are selected and dry refuse is dumped over there. When the area is filled it is leveled and covered with earth. Dumping serves two purposes, first low lying areas are filled, and secondly the levelled land may be used for agricultural purposes or otherwise. But indiscriminate dumping is a nuisance to the public since during summer and rainy season it emits very offensive gases. It acts as a breeding place for flies, attracts rodents, pigs and stray cattles who scatter the refuse adding further nuisance to the public. The air and ground water also gets polluted.

  (ii) **Controlled Tipping :** This is the best method of disposal of refuse. In this method trenches or pits of 3 feet depth but not in any case more than 6 feet in depth are dug in an open land away from the habitation. The refuse is put in the trench and covered with earth daily. When the trench is nearly full it is completely covered with earth and the trench is allowed to remain as such for a period of about 6 months. During this period certain chemical and bacteriological changes will take place and heat is produced which will convert the refuse into manure. At the end of six months when the refuse is fully decomposed, the pits are dug open and the manure is removed which is used in fields and pits are reused. The earth which is put daily as a layer over the refuse prevents the escape of gases and spread of refuse by air. Moreover flies, insects etc. will not be attracted.

When the low lying area is filled by disposal of refuse either by dumping or by controlled tipping method that must not be used for construction of buildings at least for 10 years. This land may be used for agricultural purposes.

(iii) **Burial :** Burial is another method of disposal of dry refuse when the requirement of refuse disposal is for short period of time as in camps. In this method a trench is dug and refuse is dumped in it and covered with earth daily. When the trench is full it is completely covered with earth and another trench is dug for further use.

(iv) **Compositing :** Compositing is the process of converting organic matter into manure with the help of bacterial action. This method is used in some cities and towns where refuse is disposed of along with human excreta (night soil). In this method trenches or pits of 3 feet depth are dug. Refuse and human excreta are put in the trenches in alternate layers in the proportion of 6" and 2" thickness of refuse and night soil respectively. The uppermost layer should always be of refuse. When the trenches are full they are covered with earth. After this they are left as such for about 6 months for compositing. As a result of chemical and bacterial action intense heat is produced inside the compost pits. The temperature rises to about 60°C. At this temperature the pathogenic and other micro-organisms are killed and pits gradually cool down. After 4-6 months the decomposition is complete and manure is formed which is used for agriculural purposes. The pits are reused. This method of disposal of refuse and human excreta is also known as 'Hot fermentation process'.

Mechanical Compositing : This is an advanced method of refuse disposal. In this method the water insoluble or large size substances such as rags, metal, glass, stones, bones etc. are sorted out from the refuse, then it is ground in a mechine to reduce the size of particles. This ground refuse is then mixed with sewage containing night soil, mixed well mechanically and then incubated. In this process the chemical and bacteriological decomposition takes place and entire period of compositing is complete in 4-6 weeks. The compost so formed is used as manure. Such composting plants are used in big cities.

(v) **Burning :** Burning is one of the best methods of disposing of the refuse where sufficient land for pits is not available for dumping etc. This process is also known as incineration and the equipment used for this purpose is called incinerator. Burning is more suitable for disposing of the hospital refuse which is generally more infectious than street refuse because of the presence of various types of discharges, blood and dead tissues of patients. The burning is carried out in an incinerator.

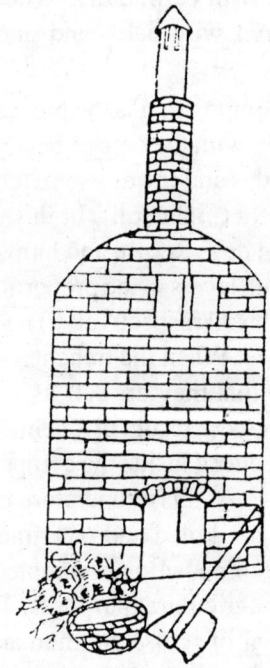

Fig. 5.8 : An incinerator.

If refuse contains pieces of glass, metal, sand etc. then they may create problems in burning which will have to be sorted out. Although burning is a good method of disposal of refuse but it has certain drawbacks :

(i) There is direct loss of manure.

(ii) It is an expensive method.

(iii) An incinerator is required.

(iv) During rainy reason this process may not be very effective due to excess content of moisture in the refuse which may not burn properly.

Refuse disposal is a very important part of environmental hygiene and public health. It is the duty of the government to make arrangements for the proper disposal of refuse. The public should be educated through different medias regarding the advantages of proper refuse disposal. The public must give full co-operation in this cause. Even if we have the most sophisticated machinery for collection and disposal of refuse, and the public does not co-operate then the whole system will fail therefore involvement of the public is very important.

Excreta Disposal

To improve the community health it is very important that the human excreta is disposed of in a sanitary manner. If excreta is disposed of hygienically the public can be protected from majority of diseases and crores of rupees can be saved which are spent every year in controlling various diseases. Human excreta is a major source of infection as it contains pathogenic micro-organisms, viruses, protozoa, helminthic parasites and their eggs. The faeces of a patient contains various disease producing agents which are transmitted to a new host through water, food, flies, contaminated fingers and soil. It directly pollutes the water and food which when ingested by a healthy person leads to the production of diseases. The diseases which are associated with improper disposal of excreta include typhoid, paratyphoid, fever, diarrhoea, dysentery, cholera, poliomyelitis, viral hepatitis, round worm and hook worm infestation etc.

In villages people go to fields for defecation and least care is paid towards the proper disposal of human excreta. That is why the incidence of above mentioned diseases are more in villages. The villagers do not have hygienic sense. The children defecate in or near the houses and flies sit over the faeces. Again they sit on the food and even milk feeders of the kids and contaminate them with faecal matter attached to their wings and legs thus easily spread the disease.

The chain of spreading the diseases can be broken easily if faecal matter is promptly disposed of in an hygienic manner. In this way the excreta will not contaminate water, food and soil and community health will improve.

For disposal of human excreta there are several methods in use. Some of which are applicable to rural and unsewered areas and others are applicable to sewered areas. For this purpose following methods are used :

(a) Rural and unsewered areas :
  (i) Service type
  (ii) Non-service type
(b) Sewered areas :
  Water carriage system and sewage treatment.

(i) Service Type of Latrines

In rural and unsewered area the disposal of human excreta is a great problem. The night soil (human excreta) is collected by manual labour from privies (structure for depositing excreta in private household) and latrines (similar structure for public use). In privies or latrines the excreta is collected in buckets or pails which are removed by sweepers and transferred to night soil carts for transportation to distant places of final disposal. This system is called service type or conservancy system and such latrines are called service type of latrines. This is an old system, though it is being discarded and replaced by water carriage system but still it is used in villages and small towns where water carriage system is not provided by the authorities due to high costs of laying down sewers and water carriage system.

Conservancy system is not a good system from health point of view and has the following drawbacks :

  (i) Night soil is exposed to flies even in carts.
  (ii) There is soil and water pollution.
  (iii) Buckets and pails are never emptied satisfactorily. Some quantity of night soil always remains sticking to the buckets.
  (iv) It gives highly objectionable smell especially when the latrines are cleaned.
  (v) Buckets and pails often get corroded and require frequent replacement which is a costly affair.
  (vi) A large number of manual labourers are required hence not economical from financial point of view.
  (vii) Above all it is against the human diginity that human beings

are employed for removing the excreta of other human beings. So the service type of latrines are discarded and discouraged and efforts are made to convert such latrines to sanitary latrines which do not require any service in its disposal.

(ii) Non-Service Type Latrines

Non-service type of latrines include :

  (a) Bore hole latrine
  (b) Dug well latrine
  (c) Water seal latrine
  (d) R.C.A. latrine, (Research Cum Action Project, Government of India).
  (e) Shallow trench latrine
  (f) Deep trench latrine

(b) Water Carriage System

Water carriage system is also known as sewerage system. In this system the human excreta is collected and removed along with waste water through underground pipes known as sewers to a distant place for final disposal. The sewage includes excreta, urine, waste water from houses, commercial establishments, factories, stables, and rain water. Water carriage system is a method of choice but it requires piped water system for flushing the latrines; there can be no sewerage system without a piped water supply. It requires lot of money to lay down the underground system of pipes and to maintain the system. This method has number of advantages that :

  (i) It requires no manual labour for removal of human excreta.
  (ii) The latrines always remain clean.
  (iii) There is no nuisance of smell or flies.
  (iv) Spreading of diseases by insects, rodents or animals is checked.
  (v) There can be overall improvement of community health.

Medical Entomology : There are a large number of arthropods present in the environment of man and they constitute the largest group among the invertebrates. Many of them are harmful, some are useful and others are of no significance. A few arthropods bite or infest man and transmit diseases. A study of these arthropods (mainly insects) is known as medical entomology. The word arthropod is derived from two words arthro means jointed and pods means legs. So the main characteristics of all arthropods is that they have many joints in their legs.

CLASSIFICATION OF ARTHROPODS

From medical point of view arthropods are classified as follows :

(i) **Class Insecta :** Insects constitute the largest group among arthropods which are intimately related to man, and they play an important part in the transmission of diseases. The body of insects is divided into three parts i.e. head, thorax and abdomen. Head has a pair of eyes, antennae and a mouth. Thorax is formed by three fused segments. To the lower surface of thorax, three pairs of legs and one or two pairs of wings (some of them without wings) are attached. The abdomen is made up of 9-11 segments, out of these last two segments form the external genitalia. The reproduction is by laying eggs. The winged insects undergo four stages of development i.e. egg, larva, pupa and adult whereas the insects without wings undergo three stages of development i.e. egg, nymph and adult. The examples of insects include mosquitoes, flies, lice and fleas.

(ii) **Class Arachnida :** They are wingless insects and the body has two parts i.e. cephalothorax and abdomen and no wings. They all have four pairs of legs and no antennae. The examples are ticks and mites.

(iii) **Class Crustacia :** The body of these is divided into two parts i.e. cephalothorax and abdomen and no wings. They have five pairs of legs and two pairs of antennae. Cyclops is the only member of this class.

Arthropod Born Diseases

Insects play an important role in the transmission of diseases. They transmit the diseases by :

1. **Direct Contact :** Some arthropods spread disease by very close personal contact, for example scabies is caused and spread by itch mite through direct contact.

2. **Mechanical Transmission :** Some arthropods carry infectious agents on their legs and wings and transfer them to the food of healthy persons thus they act as mechanical carriers. House fly is the common example of this type which spreads diarrhoea and dysentery by mechanical transmission.

3. **Biological Transmission :** Biological transmission is the most important mode of transmission. In this mode the disease agent multiplies or undergoes some developmental changes in the insect host and then carried to human host. Examples of biological transmission include malaria and filaria by mosquitoes and plague by the rat flea.

Arthropod diseases are more prevalent in warm regions than cold climates. They also occur in temperate climates at crowded and dirty places where mosquitoes and flies etc. can grow easily and rapidly. Some arthropod borne diseases are as follows :

1. MOSQUITO

Mosquitoes are small insects living in houses or near the houses. They are found all over the world. The body of the mosquito consists of three segments i.e. head, thorax and abdomen. The head is conical in shape and bears a long needle like structure called the proboscis with which the mosquito bites. The thorax has a pair of wings and three pairs of legs. When the mosquito is at rest the wings are folded. The buzzing noise of the mosquito is produced by the beating of their wings. The female mosquito bites and sucks the blood of human beings and pet animals. The male mosquito does not bite and lives on plant juices. Blood meal is necessary for producing eggs. With each bite by the

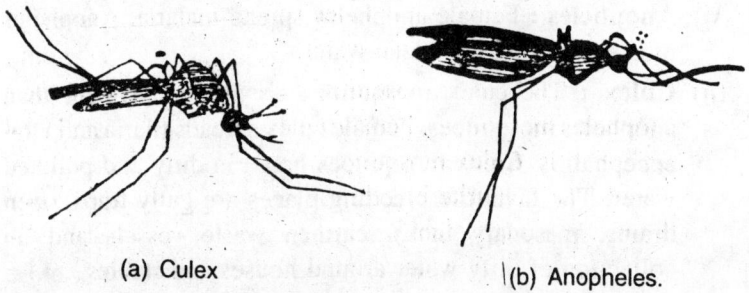

(a) Culex   (b) Anopheles.

Fig. 5.9 (a) & (b) : Mosquito

mosquito blood is sucked and a small fluid is injected in the blood which leads to itching sensation and discomfort to the person.

The female mosquito after sucking blood, lays eggs on the surface of water in wells, cisterns, fountains, water receptacles etc. In rural areas it breeds in pools, banks of streams or canals, drains or garden pits containing seepage water. They also breed in gully traps, masonary tanks and on collection of dirty water around houses and stables. During the course of season the female mosquito may lay eggs several times and 100 to 200 even more at a time. Like other insects mosquitoes also have four stages in their life cycle i.e. egg, larva, pupa and adult.

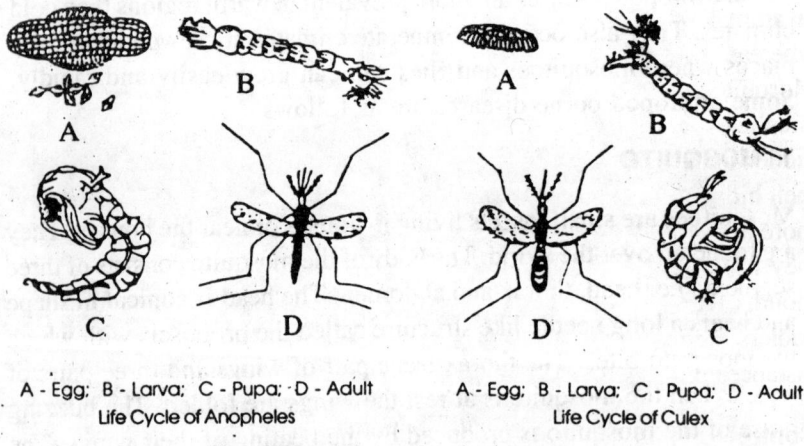

A - Egg; B - Larva; C - Pupa; D - Adult
Life Cycle of Anopheles

A - Egg; B - Larva; C - Pupa; D - Adult
Life Cycle of Culex

Fig. 5.10 : Life cycle of mosquito.

There are three main types of mosquitoes which spread the diseases. They include :

(i) **Anopheles :** Female anopheles spread malaria. Anopheles mosquitoes breed in clean water.

(ii) **Culex :** The culex mosquitoes are more prevalent than anopheles mosquitoes. Female culex spreads filaria and viral encephalitis. Culex mosquitoes breed in dirty and polluted water. The favourite breeding places are gully traps, open drains, masonary tanks, earthen waste vessels and on collection of dirty water around houses and stables.

(iii) **Aedes Mosquito :** Aedes mosquito is also known as tiger mosquito. It is generally found in houses and is characteristically marked with white stripes on a black body. Because of these stripes on their bodies they are called 'tiger mosquitoes'. The females are blood suckers and bite during day and night. These mosquitoes are most abundant during rainy season. They breed in artificial collections of water i.e. water found in broken bottles, flower pots, fire buckets etc. Aedes mosquitoes are responsible for spreading yellow fever (not present in India), dengue fever and haemorrhagic fever.

The male mosquitoes do not bite, only the female mosquitoes bite because they need blood for laying eggs. Some mosquitoes live on human blood whereas others live on animal blood. The mosquitoes which live on human blood are more dangerous than those who live on animal blood. The life of male mosquito is not more than 1-3 weeks whereas female mosquitoes may live upto 4 months or more. Mosquitoes prefer to live at dark places. Some mosquitoes like anopheles avoid heat and light therefore during day time they remain hidden in the corners, under luggage or in the shoes and come out from their hiding places at night time in search of food. In fact, they become more active after sunset and just before sunrise. After sucking blood, they usually rest on the surface of walls. During winter and hottest months the mosquitoes undergo hibernation in covered places like coolers etc. and do not breed. The mosquitoes cannot fly over long distances but may fly upto 2-3 kilometres from their breeding places.

Control of Mosquitoes

(i) Do not allow water to stagnate near the houses. Low lying areas must be filled with dust and levelled so as to eliminate the breeding places.

(ii) Sprinkle oil on the surface of water. Oil will spread easily on water and it will kill mosquito larvae and pupae partly by suffocation, drowning action and partly by its toxic action. The oils commonly used for this purpose are crude oil, kerosene oil, petrol and malariol. Sprinkling of oil on water has the drawbacks that it renders the water unfit for consumption and it may also kill the fishes.

(iii) A recent technique is that some kind of fish like Gambusia, Barbados, lebister are grown in water. The fish readily feed on mosquito larvae thus causes reduction is mosquito larvae.

(iv) Houses and cattle sheds should be sprayed with insecticides, a wide variety of which are available in the market. These insecticides include DDT, BHC, malathion etc. which are recommended for control of adult mosquitoes. These insecticides may be sprayed on the walls and roofs with an ordinary stirrup pump or still better with a compression pressure sprayer.

(v) Mosquito repellants should be used in the houses or applied on the body.

(vi) Mosquito nets should be used.

(vii) Doors, windows and ventilators of buildings should be fitted with fine gauge so that mosquitoes and other insects may not enter inside the building.

(viii) Regular cleaning of houses and unused articles should be done so as to prevent hiding of mosquitoes.

2. FLIES

Among various kinds of flies viz. house flies, sand flies, tsetse flies and black flies the most important is the house fly. There are many species of houseflies, the most common species is known as **Musca domestica**. It is a small, very common and widely distributed insect which lives close to man.

The body of house fly is divided into three segments i.e. head, thorax and abdomen. The head has a pair of antennae, a pair of compound eyes and a proboscis with which it sucks fluids. The thorax has three pairs of legs and a pair of wings. The body and legs of the house fly are densely covered with short hairs which secrete a sticky substance that helps in spreading of diseases.

A house fly does not bite therefore does no harm to a person in direct manner but otherwise they are major source of spreading the diseases. They spread the disease mechanically as they carry the pathogenic germs on body, legs and wings and frequently move from one place to another and contaminate the food of human beings and animals. The housefly has a tendency of frequent vomiting and defacating while feeding and has the habit of defacating constantly

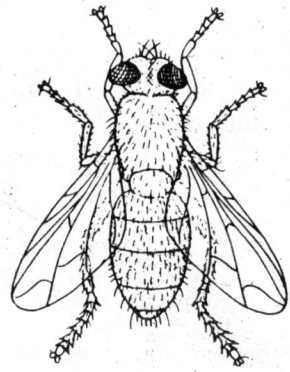

Fig. 5.11 : House fly.

throughout the day. Thus it deposits countless bacteria in the exposed food.

A house fly breeds on human excreta, cow dung, horse manure, refuse collections, decaying and fermenting vegetable and animal matter. It requires moisture for breeding therefore cannot breed in very dry materials. A female house fly lays 100-150 eggs at a time in moist decaying organic matter like human excreta, animal excreta, garbage and vegetable refuse. It lays 5 or 6 such batches of eggs in a season. The life cycle of house fly has four stages i.e. egg, larva, pupa and adult. The life cycle from egg to adult takes about 10-20 days for completion which depends on temperature. The greater the temperature and humidity, the quicker the cycle. A house fly can live for more than 15 days in summer and 25 days in winter. In autumn season they are subjected to a natural disease which kill them in large numbers.

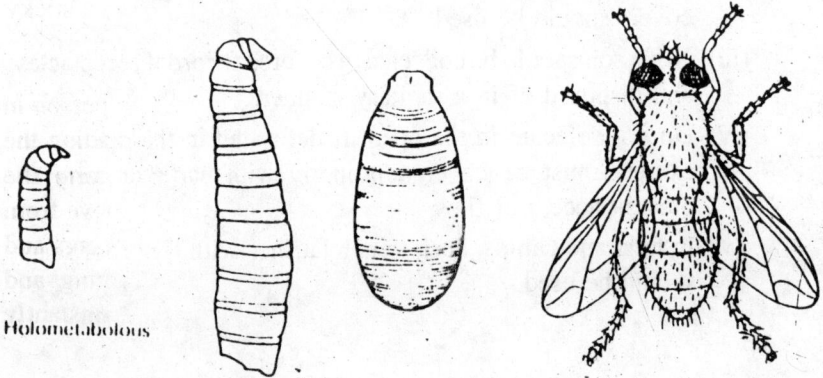

Holometabolous

Fig. 5.12 : Life cycle of house fly.

Fly Borne Diseases

Flies are responsible for spreading a large number of diseases like diarrhoea, dysentery, gastroenteritis, cholera, typhoid, paratyphoid fever, amoebiasis, trachoma, conjunctivitis, worm infestations, polio.

Control of Flies

Fly nuisance can be controlled by adopting following measures :

(a) Prevention of Breeding of Flies

(i) Promptly remove and properly dispose of human excreta, cow dung, horse manure, refuse and organic matter.

(ii) Do not allow the refuse to accumulate near the habitation specially stables, cow sheds, slaughter houses, fish markets etc. They should be regularly cleaned.

(iii) Do not throw the refuse in the open on roads or streets. Put it in the covered dust bins.

(iv) For destruction of eggs, larvae and pupae of flies in the manure apply some toxic substance to the manure. For this purpose borax, gammexane, chlorodane etc. can be used. DDT does not much have much effect on fly larvae.

(v) Keep as much cleanliness as possible.

(b) Prevention of Flies to Reach Human Excreta

(i) Human excreta should be disposed of by water carriage system.

(ii) Fly proof privies and latrines provided with self closing seat covers should be used.

(iii) Night soil should be collected in covered fly proof receptacles and disposed of in a sanitary manner.

(iv) Do not defecate in the open. If defecated in the open then excreta must be covered properly with earth or sand to prevent access of flies.

(v) In fairs and camps, deep trench latrines with fly proof seats should be used.

(c) Protection of Food from Flies

(i) The food should be protected from flies by covering it with wire-gauge or muslin cloth.

(ii) The hawkers and stall owners should cover the eatables with wire gauge, muslin cloth or should keep in glass cases, fly proof almirahs etc. specially prepared for the purpose.

(iii) The doors, windows and ventilators of houses, restaurants, hotels, confectionary stores, hospitals, fish and meat markets should be fitted with wire mesh which will give a considerable relief from house flies and prevent contamination of food by them.

(iv) Electric fans may be used to force a current of air over the food products which will prevent the flies to settle over the food products.

(d) Killing of Adult Flies

(i) Sticky fly papers, strings or tangle foot are prepared by smearing a hot mixture of castor oil and resin on glazed paper or strings. They are placed in rooms or suspended from walls. Flies stick to them and die. They are effective as long as they remain sticky. With this method only small number of flies can be reduced.

(ii) Fly traps of different varieties are available in the market. The conical hoop fly trap is most effective and economical. The bait is placed at the bottom of the cone. The flies are attracted towards it due to odour of the bait and trapped inside. Afterwards the flies are killed by fumigation.

(iii) Now a days electric insect killers are available in the market which are quite effective for killing the flies.

(iv) In small numbers flies are killed by wire mesh or hard flaps of plastic or leather fitted with handles.

(v) Poisonous baits may be used for killing the flies. The insecticides such as DDT, BHC have now become ineffective in killing the house flies largely because the flies have developed resistance to these insecticides. A poisonous bait of 2% formalin solution with little sugar and milk is placed in the rooms to attract flies, since they are thirstly insects, are always attracted towards water or the solution and die after drinking the poisonous solution.

No fly control measure will be successful unless people give full co-operation in this measure. Public should be convinced through health education that house fly is a carrier of diseases hence they must adopt anti-fly measures. It has been rightly said that a clean house with clean surroundings can lesson the fly problem to a great extent. So clean habits should be adopted. Houses, surroundings and habitations must be kept clean to decrease the insect problems.

3. LICE

They are small wingless electroparasites i.e. they are parasites which live entirely on mammalian blood outside the body of human or animal host. They are of three types :

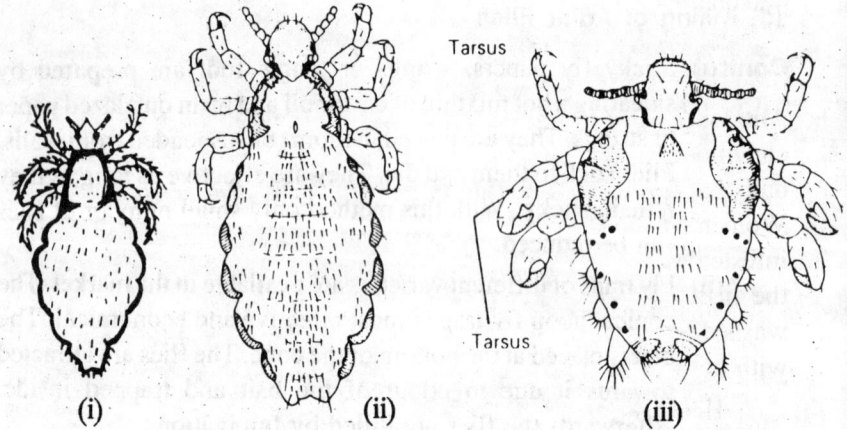

Fig 5.13 : (i) Body louse (ii) Head louse (iii) Pubic or crab louse.

(i) Head louse : Infests the hair of the head.

(ii) Body louse : It is found in the seams of clothes and beddings and hair of the chest and armpits.

(iii) Pubic or crab louse : It is found in the pubic and anal region. It adheres so close to the skin that manual removal is very difficult.

The head and body lice resemble each other and cannot be distinguished so easily whereas pubic or crab louse can be distinguished easily by its small and square body with powerful legs and claws.

The body of louse is divided into three parts i.e. head, thorax and abdomen. The head has sucking type of mouth parts, the thorax has three pairs of legs, the abdomen is divided into segments. They suck the mammalian blood throughout their life and breed on the body, hair or clothes of the host. Life cycle of louse has three stages i.e. egg, larva and adult. The average life of a louse is from 35 to 58 days. Infection is by direct contact through combs, brushes, clothings etc. Both male and female lice are blood suckers. They are attached to the host firmly for frequent blood feeds and it is difficult to remove them manually.

Louse Borne Diseases

Louse borne diseases are typhus, relapsing fever and trench fever. Head lice may lead to swollen glands at the back of the neck and ears. The bites of louse are irritating, causing disturbed and insufficient sleep especially in children. Louse infestations are generally due to poor personal hygiene of the host.

Control of Lice

Anti louse measures include improvement in personal hygiene, general cleanliness of the body, hair, clothes and other household articles. A daily bath with soap and water is essential to limit the louse infestation. Women with long hair should wash and clean their hair frequently. Hair infested with lice must be combed with a thick comb so as to remove the lice from hair. The clothings, towels and bed sheets should be washed with soap and hot water and after drying they should be pressed with hot iron. Highly infested clothings should be autoclaved.

Head louse can be quickly controlled if 1 percent DDT dust is applied to hair and after 24 hours the hair is washed thoroughly, dried and combed with a thick comb. A second application may be repeated after one week. 0.2 percent lindane (gamma-BHC) dissolved in coconut oil can also be used for this purpose. Pubic parts and armpits must be cleaned regularly and hair should be cut short.

4. FLEAS

Fleas are wingless insects, 2-3 mm long with laterally compressed hard body consisting of three segments i.e. head, thorax and abdomen. A flea has 3 pairs of legs attached to the thorax. The life cycle has four stages i.e. egg, larva, pupa, adult. There are large varieties of fleas like rat flea, cat flea, dog flea. Rat flea is an important member of this group because they transmit the dreaded disease, plague. Generally fleas live on rodents. In the absence of rats when they are starved they bite man. Both male and female fleas bite man and suck blood. Fleas transmit disease by biting. The bite of a hungry flea is particularly dangerous because it is sure to inject plague bacilli in the human beings. The flea borne diseases are :

   (i) Bubonic plague

  (ii) Endemic typhus

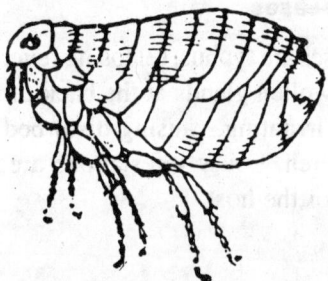

Fig. 5.14 : Rat flea.

Control of Fleas

    (i) Eliminate rats and other rodents. When the rodents are eliminated fleas will also be controlled.

   (ii) Pet animals like cats and dogs should be dusted with 10 percent DDT.

  (iii) Insecticides like 10% DDT or 5% malathion must be dusted over rat runs, under carpets, gunny bags and other hiding places.

  (iv) 10% DDT or 5% malathion must also be blown into rat holes with the help of dust blower.

   (v) Improve sanitary conditions in the house as well as in the surroundings so that the rodents do not find hiding places.

5. TICKS

Ticks are ectoparasites of vertebrates. They are small insects and their body is not distinctly separated into head, thorax and abdomen. They have four pairs of legs and no antennae. Their life cycle has four stages i.e. egg, larva, nymph and adult.

Ticks are found is warm climate and are nocturnal in habit. They either live on the body of the hosts like dogs, cats and cattle or in the cracks of the walls and floor and come out in the night for blood sucking. Both male and female bite and suck the blood. The female tick may remain attached to its host for a longer period but male usually drops off after a few days. Sometimes they attack man and transmit diseases. There are two types of ticks i.e. hard ticks and soft ticks.

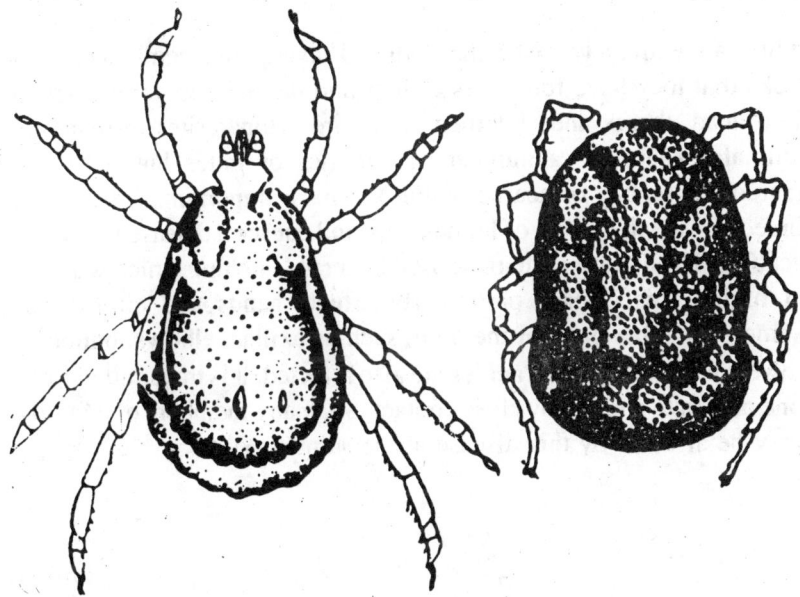

Fig 5.15 : Ticks—Hard & Soft.

Hard tick is so called because the dorsum of its body is covered by a hard shield called scutum. The soft tick does not have this hard dorsal shield and its head is situated ventrally which is not seen from above. This makes it easy to identify a soft tick from a hard tick.

Hard tick transmits tick typhus, viral encephalitis, haemorrhagic fever and soft tick transmits relapsing fever.

Control of Ticks

(i) DDT, lindane or malathion should be sprayed in the tick infested area.

(ii) Animals like dogs, cats and cattle should be dusted with DDT or malathion.

    (iii) Cracks in the floor and walls should be filled up.

    (iv) Workers handling the animals should protect themselves from ticks by wearing protective clothings and taking other precautions so that ticks do not attach to their bodies. If any tick is found on the body that must be removed immediately and killed.

6. MITES

Mites are extremely small arthropods and have quite resemblance with ticks that they have four pairs of legs and the body is not demarked into head, thorax and abdomen. They are ectoparasites to man and animals. There are a number of varieties of mites but itch mite (sarcoptes scabiei or acarus scabiei) is most important. It lives and breeds inside the layers of human skin and causes a disease known as scabies. The disease is characterised by terrible itching which worsens at night. This disease particularly affects hands and elbows but sometimes other parts of the body such as axillae, elbows, buttocks, lower abdomen, feet and ankles are also affected. It is transmitted from one person to another by close contact. So, many members of a family may be affected by this disease at the same time.

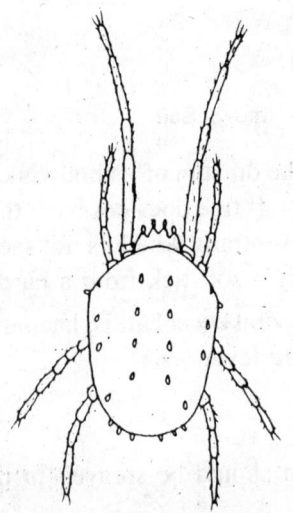

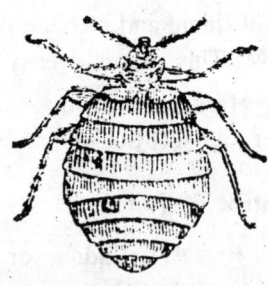

Fig. 5.16 : Itch mites.   **Fig. 5.17 :** Bed bug (dorsal view).

Control of Scabies

  (i) For prevention avoid over crowding and maintain personal cleanliness and hygiene.

  (ii) Treat all the affected persons of the family. They should be bathed thoroughly with soap and water and then apply one of the following medicaments on the body which should be washed next day and the course repeated as suggested by the physician. The medicaments used for scabies are :

    (a) Benzyl benzoate 25% emulsion;

    (b) Sulphur ointment 2 to 10%; and

    (c) Benzene hexachloride 0.5% in coconut oil.

7. BED BUG

It is small, thin dark brown insect. It measures 3 to 5 mm in length and 1.5 to 2.5 mm in breadth. The head is short and broad having a pair of compound eyes and a pair of antannae. Both male and female bugs bite with their strong beak causing a painful wound. They prefer human blood and in its absence feed on blood of rats and domestic animals. It is nocturnal in habits. During day time they remain hidden in cracks of furniture, cracks in the walls etc. and come out at night for feeding. After biting they inject an irritating fluid to the body which causes a flow of blood to the spot and causes local inflammation. A bed bug can live upto one year even without food.

Bed bugs do not directly transmit any disease but they cause irritation, local inflammation, annoyance and loss of sleep. Bed bugs can be controlled by spraying gammaxane, D.D.T. or kerosene oil containing pyrethrum in the bed bug infested areas. They are killed by pouring boiling water in the cracks of furniture and floors. The cracks in floor and walls should be permanently sealed.

8. CYCLOPS

Cyclop or water flea is a small transparent insect found in fresh water. It swims on water with characteristic jerky movements. They are visible to the naked eye and can be easily strained or killed by boiling. It is the intermediate host of guinea worm disease. Man gets infection by drinking water contaminated with cyclops.

Rodents

Rodents live in close proximity of man and cause a great damage not only to buildings, crops, food stuffs and other items but also transmit very serious diseases to man like plague therefore they must be destroyed and eliminated by using the following methods :

    (i) Trapping

    (ii) Using rat poisons or rodenticides

    (iii) Fumigating the rat burrows

    (iv) Improving the sanitation

There are two types of rodents i.e. domestic and wild. The common example of domestic rodent is house rat and sewer rat. There are large varieties of wild rodents. They damage the food crops, fertile land and banks of water channels by making burrows over there.

The rodents spread a large number of diseases like plague, rat bite fever, leptospirosis, salmonellosis, haemorrhagic fever, encephalitis, scrub typhus, amoebiasis etc.

6

MICROBIOLOGY

Microbiology is a branch of science which deals with propagation, isolation and identification of micro-organisms. The causative agents of communicable diseases are very minute which are not visible to the naked eye because human eye cannot see objects less than 100 nm in size so they can be seen either with magnifying lens or with a compound microscope. Some of the micro-organisms are too small that they cannot be seen even with compound microscope so these types of micro-organisms can be seen only with an electron microscope developed by Ruslka in 1934. Such micro-organisms were called viruses. Most viruses are less than 0.2 µm in diameter.

All micro-organisms are not harmful to man. Most of them are useful which are known as non-pathogenic and only a small fraction of them are capable of producing diseases in man which are known as pathogenic (disease producing). The pathogenic micro-organisms may attack the human body and produce infection. The diseases so spread are known as communicable diseases.

Classification

Various disease producing micro-organisms are classified as follows:

1. Bacteria
2. Algae
3. Fungi, moulds and yeasts
4. Rickettsias

5. Mycoplasmas

6. Viruses

7. Protozoa

Micro-organisms may also be classified as :

(i) **Prokaryotic :** Micro-organisms with relatively smaller and simpler form of cells are known as prokaryotic microorganisms which include bacteria, rickettsias and mycoplasmas.

(ii) **Eukaryotic :** Micro-organisms with well developed cell structures are known as eukaryotic micro-organisms which include algae, fungi, moulds and protozoa.

1. BACTERIA

Bacteria is a unicellular micro-organism which does not contain chlorophyll. The common pathogenic bacteria generally vary in size from 0.2 to 1.5 μ in diameter and 3 to 14 μ in length. They reproduce by an asexual process, characteristically by simple cell division. They grow and reproduce when favourable conditions are available. They are present everywhere i.e. air, water, soil, internal and external parts of the human body, animals and plants.

All bacteria are not harmful, many of them are very useful such as in the preparation of curd and cheese. They are also useful in the preparation of wine and in the synthesis of certain vitamins in the body. A number of bacteria are used for preparing antibiotics. Some bacterias like nitrogen fixing bacteria are helpful for the growth of plants. Pathogenic bacteria are responsible for causing many diseases in man and animals.

Classification

Bacteria are classified according to their shapes which are given below:

(i) Cocci	Oval or spiral shaped
(ii) Bacilli	Rod shaped
(iii) Vibrios	Comma shaped
(iv) Spirilla	Spiral shaped
(v) Spirochaetes	Spiral shaped cells which look like coiled hairs.

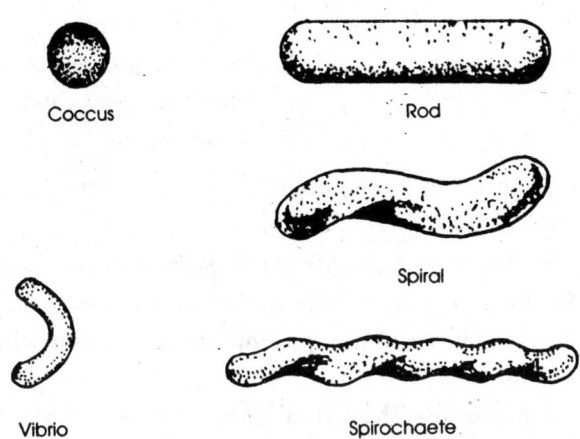

Coccus

Rod

Spiral

Vibrio

Spirochaete

Fig. 6.1 : Different shapes of bacteria.

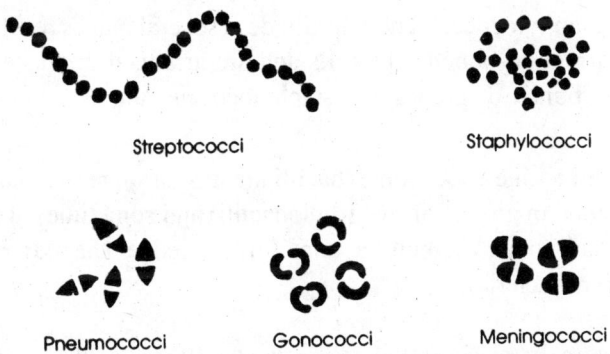

Streptococci

Staphylococci

Pneumococci

Gonococci

Meningococci

Fig. 6.2 : Different Types of Cocci.

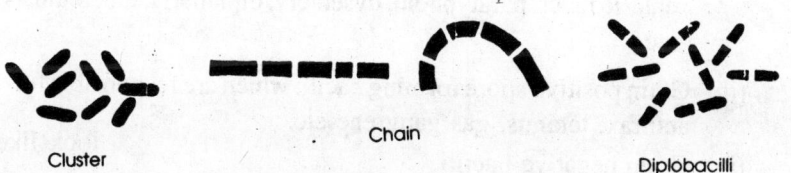

Cluster

Chain

Diplobacilli

Fig. 6.3 : Different Types of Bacilli.

    (vi) Actinomycetes   Branching filamentous bacteria. They are so called because they resemble with rays of the sun.

   (vii) Mycoplasma   They are without a cell wall and occur as round or oval bodies or as interlacing filaments.

A. Depending on their characteristic arrangements, bacteria may further be classified as follows :

  (a) Micrococci – The cells are arranged singly or irregularly.

  (b) Diplococci – The cells divide in one plane and remain attached in pairs e.g. pneumococcus, meningococcus and gonococcus.

  (c) Streptococci – The cells divide in one plane and are arranged in chains of different length e.g. streptococcus pyogens.

  (d) Tetracocci – The cells divide in two planes at right angles to one another and form groups of four. They very rarely produce diseases in human beings.

  (e) Staphylococci – The cells divide is several planes resulting in irregular bunches of cells and are arranged in clusters like a bunch of grapes e.g. staphylococcus aureus.

B. **Bacilli :** Like cocci some bacilli are also arranged in chains, in clusters, in groups of two (diplobacilli) and sometimes at angles to each other making a cuneiform (wedge shaped) pattern (corynebacteria).

According to staining reactions the bacilli are further classified as:

  (i) Acid fast bacilli.

  (ii) Gram positive non-sporing bacilli which are responsible for enteric fever, paratyphoid, dysentery, diphtheria, tuberculosis etc.

 (iii) Gram positive spore forming bacilli which are responsible for anthrax, tetanus, gas gangrene etc.

 (iv) Gram negative bacilli.

Some bacteria (bacilli and clostridium) have the ability to form endospores, usually one in each bacterial cell which are always resting spores. They can withstand very unfavourable conditions such as very high temperature, extreme dryness, freezing, treatment with very poisonous chemicals etc. for months or even several years. However these spores are destroyed by autoclaving at 120°C for 15 minutes. Bacteria cannot multiply under these conditions but whenever favourable conditions are available the spores germinate into bacterial cells.

Structure of Bacterial Cell

Bacteria are not properly visible under compound microscope but they can be properly and clearly seen under electron microscope. The bacterial cell structure as seen under electron microscope is described below.

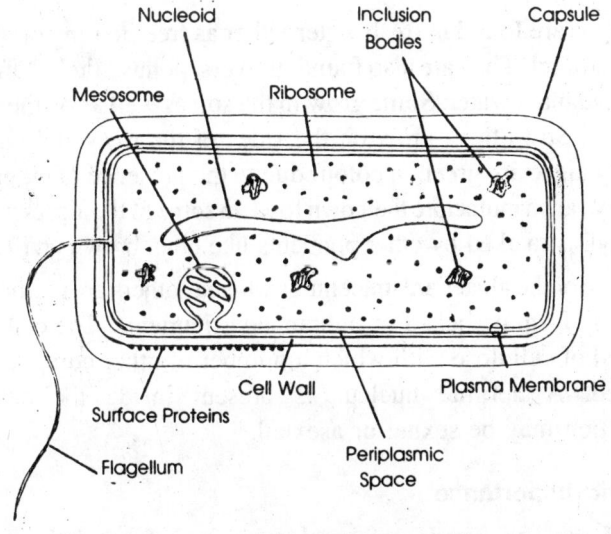

Fig. 6.4 : Structure of Bacterial Cell.

The structure of an ideal bacterial cell consists of distinct but complex cell wall made of proteins and carbohydrates. The cell wall is surrounded with a distinct sheath or capsule. The capsulated form is very resistant to adverse conditions and such a condition is commonly the cause of a disease. Inside the cell wall there is a thin plasma membrane formed by the cytoplasm. The cytoplasm spreads uniformly throughout the cell which include ribosomes, mesosomes, granules, vacuoles and the nuclear body. In addition to these essential components some bacteria may contain additional structures. Several types of bacteria possess whip-like threads called flagella which originate from cytoplasm. They act as organ of locomotion. The bacteria do not possess an organised nucleus as is found in higher plants; nucleolus and nuclear membrane are absent however a nuclear material (or chromatin) is present in the bacterial cell in the form of one or two deeply staining bodies possibly representing chromosomes. Chemically these bodies are composed of twisted and folded strands of DNA (deoxyribonucleic acid) which is the genetic material of the bacterial cell. The DNA bodies divide before the division of bacterial cell and are distributed equally among the freshly divided cells.

2. ALGAE

Green algae are found in fresh water either as free floating or attached to some support. They are also found in rivers, ponds, ditches and other pools of stagnant water. Some grow in the soil as well as on the surface of the soil. Still others grow on the sides of the trees and on rocks. Generally algae are green in colour due to the presence of chlorophyll hence they can manufacture their own food. In some of the algaes the green chlorophyll is marked by other pigments like blue, brown and red.

Some of the algaes are unicellular whereas others are multicellular, which may form branched or unbranched filaments. The cell wall is composed of cellulose with which a number of other compounds are associated. A definite nucleus is present inside the cell. The reproduction may be sexual or asexual.

Economic Importance

Many of the sea weeds are used as human food, being rich in carbohydrates and vitamins. They form an important food for fish and other water animals. Brown algae called kelps are an important source of iodine. Some sea weeds are used as fertilizers because they are rich in potassium and other mineral matters. Some red algae are a rich source of agar-agar which is used in many industries including medicines. Big deposits of diatoms in sea-beds known as diatomaceous earth are available which is used in tooth powder, heat insulators and metal polishing. Though algaes have a number of advantages but some of them are a nuisance to water reservoirs as they pollute water specially in summer rains.

3. FUNGI, MOULDS AND YEASTS

Fungi constitute the largest group of thallophyta. They do not contain chlorophyll therefore they cannot manufacture their own food hence act as parasites or saprophytes for getting their nourishment.

They are unicellular or multicellular micro-organisms. They have rigid cell wall containing polysaccharides. The cytoplasmic membrane of fungi contain steroles. Their nuclei contain nuclear membrane and paired chromosomes. They reproduce sexually, asexually or by both mechanisms.

The vegetative body or thalus of algae is the mycelium which is formed of numerous, slender, thread-like colourless filaments known as hyphae. The hyphae may sometimes be woven together so as to form a false parenchymatus tissue.

Mucor

These are commonly known as pin-moulds. It is a very common fungus of saprophytic nature. It grows on moist bread, rotten fruits, decaying vegetables, shed flowers, animal dung, leather goods, wet shoes and other organic media, spreading like a cob-web. They can be easily grown on moist bread kept in a warm place for three to four days.

The body of moulds is composed of a mass of white, delicate, cotton-like threads collectively known as mycellium. Each individual thread of the mycellium is known as lypha. They commonly reproduce by asexual process and sometimes by sexual process.

Yeasts

Yeasts are the simplest, unicellular fungi. They are spherical or elliptical in shape. They produce spores by a process called 'budding' the cells produce hypha and multicellular fungi consist of haphae collectively known as mycellium. Yeast-like fungi do not form mycellium they partly grow as yeasts and partly as long filaments. The common example of pathogenic yeast like fungus is Candida albicans.

The fungi that grow either as filaments or as yeasts according to the conditions of growth are called dimorphic fungi. Most of the systemic fungal infections are caused by dimorphic fungi e.g. blastomycosis and coccidioidomycosis.

Fungal infections are very common in man and animals. Ring worm, ear and lung infections are very common in man. Fungal infections range from mild to serious and fatal. Food poisoning due to infections of certain poisonous fungi are also quite common. They spoil the food and other usuable items like leather goods, shoes, books and papers, cotton clothes etc.

The pathogenic fungi include dermatophytes, Candida albicans, cladosporium, dermatophytes, blastomyces dermatidis, histoplasma capsulatum etc.

4. RICKETTSIAS

These are simple, unicellular, gram negative microorganisms. They may be rod shaped, spherical or pleomorphic in shape. According to their properties rickettsiae are intermediate between bacteria and viruses. They differ from viruses in many ways including chemical, metabolic, reproductive and structural differences. They are parasites which can grow only in living tissues. They cannot be grown on laboratory media but can be cultivated on tissue culture media. They have typical cell wall and reproduce by asexual process i.e. fission. Chemically rickettsia contain proteins, nucleoproteins, carbohydrates, lipids and enzymes.

Pathogenic rickettsia invade different species of animals and man. The diseases caused by rickettsiae are known as rickettsiosis. Typhus fever and related diseases are caused by rickettsiae.

5. MYCOPLASMAS

Mycoplasmas are the smallest micro-organisms. The cell size ranges from 0.15 to 1 μm in diameter. Thus in size, mycoplasmas appears to be even smaller than some viruses.

Since they do not possess a true cell wall, thus they are characterised by a marked pleomorphism. They give rise to coccoid, granular, filamentous, cluster like, ring shaped, filtrable forms etc. Pleomorphism is observed in cultures and in the bodies of man and animals. They are also found in the soil, and drainage water. The diseases caused by different mycoplasmas include primary atypical pneumonia and genital infections. Besides these diseases mycoplasmas are also associated with urethritis, cervicitis, vaginitis, infertility, abortion, post partum fever and pelvic inflammatory disease.

6. VIRUSES

The name virus literally means 'poison'. They are the simplest and smallest organisms. They are very much smaller than bacteria. They vary in size from 20 nm to 300 nm (nm nanometre, 1 nm = 10^{-9}m). They cannot be seen even under high power compound microscope. However they can be seen under an electron microscope. The viruses vary in shape. Most viruses are spherical (influenza virus), rod shaped (tobacco virus), bullet shaped (rabies virus) and brick shaped (pox virus).

A virus is composed of nucleic acid DNA or RNA but never both, and a protein wall containing enzyme systems, with the help of which the virus penetrates into tissue cells. The cell wall or the special surface membrane has been named a capsid as it is composed of a certain amount of capsomers.

Viruses have no metabolic machinery of their own. They cannot synthesize their own protein and nucleic acid and hence cannot grow even on the most nutritions media. So they are strictly parasitic in nature. All forms of life, animal, plant and even bacterial are susceptible to infection by virus. The viruses which attack bacteria and destroy their nuclear material are called bacteriophages.

Many species of viruses are pathogenic for man and cause diseases ranging from common cold to highly fatal diseases such as AIDS, cancer, rabies or yellow fever. The other common diseases caused by viruses in human beings are smallpox, rabies, influenza, measlis, encephalitis, hepatitis, poliomyelitis, foot and mouth disease etc.

7. PROTOZOA

The word protozoa is derived from Greek words, protos – first and zoon—animal. They are the lowest and simplest form of animal life.

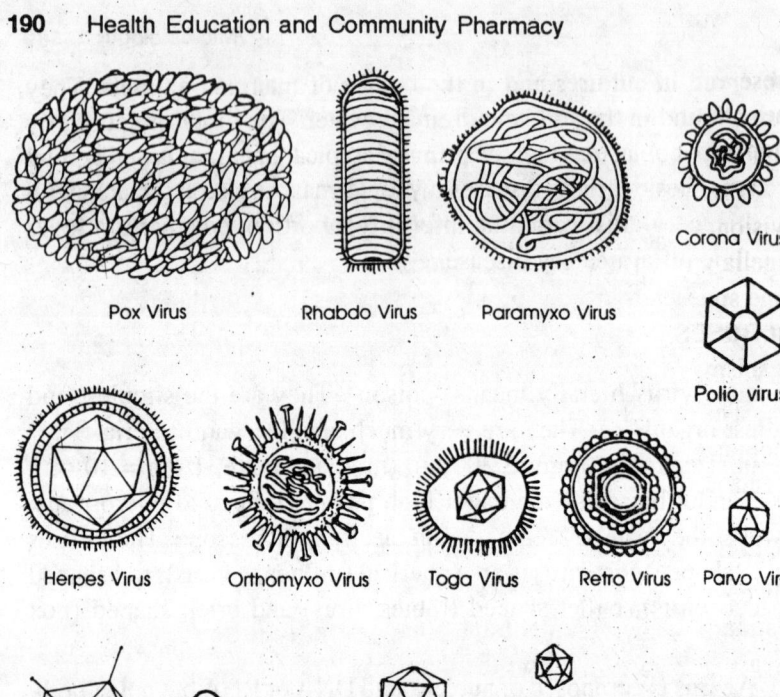

Pox Virus   Rhabdo Virus   Paramyxo Virus   Corona Virus

Herpes Virus   Orthomyxo Virus   Toga Virus   Retro Virus   Parvo Virus   Polio virus

Adeno Virus   Tobacco mosaic virus   Bacteriophage   Picorna Virus   Mumps virus

Fig. 6.5 : Comparative Sizes and Shapes of Different Viruses.

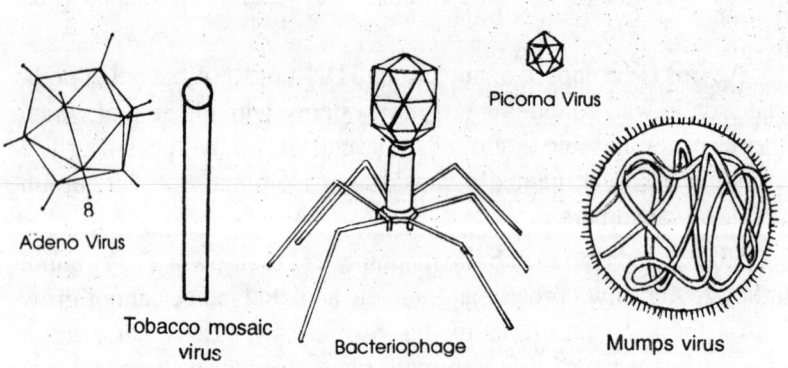

Envelope

Capsid { Capsomere

Nucleic Acid

Fig. 6.6 : Virus.

These are unicellular organisms more lightly organised than bacteria. They have protoplasm clearly differentiated into a nucleus and cytoplasm.

Protozoa reproduce by sexually, asexually, simple and multiple division. The organism moves with the help of pseudopodia, cilia, flagella and undulating membranes. Under unfavourable conditions, some species of protozoa may form round, thick walled resting cells or cysts which are more resistant forms for survival and spread of the organism.

The important human protozoal infections include malaria, amobiasis, trypanosomiasis, leishmaniasis, trichomoniasis, lambliasis, giardiasis, balantidiasis, tonoplasmosis etc.

ISOLATION OF MICRO-ORGANISMS

Whenever a patient suffering from any disease comes to a doctor for treatment, the most important point for a doctor is to diagnose the disease which is based on the detailed case history, careful physical examination and thorough laboratory investigations. Laboratory investigations are carried out in all kinds of diseases but they are extremely important in communicable diseases. For proper diagnosis of various infectious diseases it is necessary to know the type and nature of causative organism. Then and only then proper treatment with selective antibacterial agents and other drugs, route of administration, dose and duration of drug therapy can be given for early cure.

For laboratory tests specimens of possible infected material are collected. The specimens collected for testing include midstream urine, stool, blood, pus, sputum, swabs, cerebrospinal fluid (CSF), peritoneal fluid and aspiration material. One or more than one type of specimen may be collected at one time which may be repeated as suggested by the physician. The selection of correct specimen is very very important in accurate diagnosis of the disease. The specimen should be collected before giving the antimicrobial treatment otherwise the specimen may become sterile. The material collected for specimens should be from the site most likely to be infected by the suspected microorganisms. For example in urinary tract infections midstream urine sample, in fever blood samples, in diarrhoea stool sample, in respiratory tract infection sputum sample, pus sample from suppurative lesion, swab from infected areas i.e. nose, throat, ear, conjunctiva, cerebrospinal fluid in meningitis, a specimen of fresh discharge from the urethra in gonorrhoea and other sexually transmitted diseases, aspiration from different affected organs etc. should be collected in sufficient quantity in sterilized container which should be closéd with a screw cap or with sterile cotton. The container should be labelled properly and correctly. It should be sent to the laboratory as early as possible.

Isolation of Pure Culture

For studying the morphological characteristics of pathogenic micro-organism of a particular disease it is very important to get a pure culture. The growth of micro-organism in or on a laboratory medium is known as culture. When micro-organisms are grown on a solid medium from a single cell or spore it is called 'colony'. When a culture contains only one type of microbes it is termed as 'pure culture' but when it contains several species it is known as 'mixed culture'. It is very difficult to obtain a pure culture of bacteria because generally they exist as mixed cultures. But for studying the morphological characteristics of bacteria it is extremely important to have pure culture of an organism. The pure culture of micro-organisms can be obtained by growing an aliquot portion of the specimen containing bacteria on a suitable culture media which include:

    (a) nutrient broth
    (b) nutrient agar
    (c) semisolid agar
    (d) peptone water
    (e) blood agar
    (f) chocolate agar
    (g) serum agar

For the isolation of pure bacterial culture a number of methods like

1. direct transfer technique
2. single cell isolation technique
3. streak plate technique
4. serial dilution technique
5. pour plate technique etc. are used but generally pour plate technique is used.

Pour Plate Technique

The specimen containing the bacteria is first diluted in tubes of agar medium a number of times so as to get well isolated colonies of bacteria. The petriplates are thoroughly cleaned and sterilized. The agar medium is maintained at a temperature of about 42°C so as to keep it in the liquid state. The inoculum is added to this medium and shaken thoroughly so as to distribute the inoculum in the medium. The inoculated material is poured into previously cleaned and sterilized petriplates under aseptic conditions. Allow the material to cool and set. Then keep the petriplates in the incubator usually at a temperature of 37°C for 24 hours. Within this time the bacterial colonies will develop. Remove the petriplates from the incubator and watch the bacterial colonies which will be usually from single cell and are pure cultures. If the colonies are of mixed culture they may be further grown on agar plate, agar slants or on nutrient broth.

(a) Colonies on Agar Media

The bacterial culture is mixed with sterilized agar media which has been maintained at a temperature of 42°C to keep it in the liquid state. The mixture is transferred under aseptic conditions to sterilized petriplates. Allow the petriplates to incubate at a temperature of about 37°C for 24 hours. After 24 hours remove the petriplates from the incubator. The bacterial colonies of single cell or pure culture will appear on the surface of agar medium.

(b) Colonies on Agar Slants

Agar slants are prepared by putting the molten agar in sterilized test tubes. The mouth of the test tube is covered with sterilized cotton, then they are kept in a slanting position to set the medium. The surface of the medium is inoculated with bacterial culture by streaking the slanting surface of the medium in the tube with a stroke of an inoculating needle. Then the tubes are incubated at a temperature of 37°C for 24 hours.

(c) Colonies in Nutrient Broth

The sterilized nutrient broth is transferred to sterilized tubes which are then inoculated with the help of a transferring needle or loop. The tubes are then incubated at a temperature of about 37°C for 24 hours.

The colonies so developed will be pure cultures and it will be easy to study various morphological characteristics of isolated micro-organisms.

Staining of Micro-organisms

After the isolation of causative micro-organism from the infected tissue, its morphological study is carried out. For this purpose compound microscope is used. Since bacterial protoplasm has almost the same refractive index as the medium in which it grows, therefore the micro-organisms are not easily observed under the microscope but if they are stained prior to their examination then they are seen more clearly and can be easily differentiated. Therefore staining of micro-organisms prior to microscopic examination is of primary importance for the recognition of bacteria.

Stains are dyes or reagents used for colouring bacteria or other micro-organisms in order to observe them more clearly and specifically under the microscope. Various types of staining solutions commonly used in microbiology include crystal violet, methylene blue, fuchsin and safranin.

DIFFERENT STAINING TECHNIQUES

Preparation of Film or Smear

The preparation of film or smear is the first step in routine staining procedures. Film is usually prepared on 3" × 1" glass slide or sometimes on cover slip. It is essential that the glass slide or cover slip should be thoroughly clean, dry and grease free otherwise the film will not be uniform.

For ordinary use wash the slide with soap and water, dry it with a clean dry cotton cloth and then hold it with forceps and pass it through bunsen's flame 6-12 times so as make the slide free from grease. Cover slips are cleaned by dipping in chromate sulphuric acid solution, then they are first washed with tap water and then with distilled water and stored in stoppered jar in 50% alcohol.

A film is prepared by keeping a loopful of fluid material on the surface of glass slide which is spread thinly on the slide. The film is dried in the air and then fixed by passing through a bunsen's flame gently. In the bacterial culture on agar, a loopful clean water is placed on the slide with a sterilized loop. Then a minute quantity of bacterial colony is transferred to the drop with a loop and thoroughly emulsified.

The mixture is then spread uniformly as a thin film on the slide. The film is dried in the air and then heat fixed by passing through bunsen's flame gently.

STAINING TECHNIQUES

For staining the bacterial slides the following techniques are used :

A. Simple Staining

When the staining solution contains only one dye dissolved in either dilute alcohol solution or water then the stains are known as simple stains and the process is known as simple staining. Simple staining is also known as 'monochrome staining'. The dyes commonly used for simple stains include crystal violet, methylene blue, fuchsin and safranin.

Simple staining is used to study the size, shape, motility and other morphological characteristics of micro-organisms. In this type of staining, the simple stain is applied to the heat fixed film and allowed to react for 30 seconds to 3 minutes (depending on the type of stain used). Then the smear is washed with water and dried. Bacterial cells will take up the colour of the dye which will make the identification easier. Examine the slide under oil emersion lens of the microscope either directly or after mounting in glycerin.

B. Differential Staining Methods

In differential staining methods more than one dye is used which when properly employed will differentiate nearly all types of bacteria. These methods are also used to study the morphological characteristics of bacterial cells, spores and capsules. The various stains used for differential staining are Gram, crystal violet, methyl violet, fuchsin and Ziehl-Neelsen. The various staining methods used for differential staining include :

    (i) Gram's staining method
    (ii) Acid fast staining technique
    (iii) Ziehl-Neelsen method
    (iv) Staining of spores
    (v) Staining of capsules

(i) Gram's Staining Method

This is the most commonly used method for differential staining of bacteria. It is a very simple and useful method which was first used in 1884 by Gram and till now it has not lost its practical significance. All bacteria stained by Gram method can be grouped according to colour as gram positive and gram negative. The procedure for staining is as follows :

Reagents Used in Gram's Staining

(a) Gentian violet   0.5 gm.
     Distilled water upto   100 ml.
     Dissolve in distilled water.
(b) Iodine   1.0 gm.
     Potassium iodide   2.0 gm.
     Distilled water upto   100 ml.

   Dissolve potassium iodide in water and to this dissolve iodine. Add sufficient water to make up the volume to 100 ml. Store the solution in amber coloured glass bottles.

(c) Basic fuchsin   0.1 gm.
     Alcohol   10.0 ml.
     Distilled water upto   100 ml.

Dissolve basic fuchsin in alcohol and allow to stand for 24 hours. Add sufficient distilled water to make up the volume to 100 ml.

Procedure

(a) As described earlier prepare a thin film or smear of a test bacterium on a clean slide using aseptic precautions.
(b) Heat fix the film by passing through bunsen's flame 2-3 times. If heat fixation is contraindicated then dip the film in alcohol for fixation. Heat fixation coagulates the proteins of bacteria which disturbs the morphological characters of micro-organisms.
(c) Cover the fixed smear with gentian violet (crystal violet or methyl violet) stain and allow the stain to act for about one minute.
(d) Remove the excess stain and wash the slide with excess of Gram's iodine solution thoroughly.
(e) Cover the whole slide with fresh Gram's iodine solution and leave it as such for one minute. During this time compounds are formed

in the cytoplasm of the bacterial cell, which are retained by some bacterial species during decoloration with alcohol.

(f) Wash the slide with alcohol or acetone in order to decolorise the slide. Go on washing the slide till no colour comes out. This process is very rapid and completes in 2-3 seconds.

(g) After this process wash the slide under running tap water and counterstain it with an aqueous solution of fuchsin for 30 seconds.

(h) Wash the slide with tap water, dry it and examine the slide under oil immersion lens without mounting.

Those bacteria which cannot be decolorised with alcohol or acetone and retain violet colour are known as gram positive bacteria and those bacteria which are decolorised by alcohol or acetone and stains red due to fuchsin solution are known as gram negative bacteria.

The examples of gram positive bacteria are staphylococci, streptococci, pneumococci, C. diphtheriae, B. anthrasis, subtilus, Cl. tetani, Cl. welchi etc. The examples of gram negative bacteria are gonococci, meningococci, E. coli, S. typhi, Cholera vibrio etc.

The Gram staining method is commonly used for the identification of mycobacterium, streptococci, staphylococci, gonococci, E. coli etc. but this method cannot be applied to capsules, spores, flagella, fungi and protozoa. For this purpose other techniques are used which are described under respective categories.

(ii) Acid Fast Staining Technique

Acid fast staining technique was first developed by Paul Ehrlich in 1882 for differential staining of microorganisms. In this method dyes like melachite green and methylene blue are used. When the smears are treated with these dyes and washed with acids and alcohols they are not decolorised and retain the stain of the dye. Such bacteria which are not decolorised are known as acid fast bacteria but the bacteria which lose the stain and get decolorised are known as non-acid fast bacteria.

(iii) Ziehl-Neelsen Method

The Ziehl-Neelson method is used for differentiating acid fast bacteria (mycobacterium tuberculosis, a causative organism of tuberculosis and mycobacterium leprae, a causative organism of leprosy) which stain with difficulty due to their structure and hence steaming concentrated carbol fuchsin is used to stain them. The reagents used for Ziehl-Neelsen staining are :

A. Ziehl-Neelsen's (strong) carbol fuchsin solution :

    Basic fuchsin   10 gm.

    Absolute alcohol   100 ml.

    5% solution of phenol in waterupto 1000 ml.

    Dissolve basic fuchsin in alcohol and add to the phenol solution.

B. Sulphuric acid 20% solution.

C. Alcohol 95%

D. Counterstain methylene blue or malachite green.

Procedure

(a) As described earlier prepare a smear of the sputum on a slide and fix it by passing through bunsen's flame.

(b) Cover the slide with strong carbol fuchsin solution and heat until steam rises. Allow the stain to remain in contact for 5 minutes, heat being applied at intervals to keep the stain hot but the stain must not be allowed to evaporate to dryness.

(c) Wash the smear with water.

(d) Cover the slide with 20% sulphuric acid for one minute and remove excess of the acid.

(e) Wash the slide with water till the colour of the smear ceases to come out.

(f) Counterstain the slide with methylene blue or dilute malachite green for 30 seconds.

(g) Wash the slide thoroughly with water, dry it and see under oil immersion lens.

The slide will appear pink coloured and rod shaped tubercle bacilli will be seen scattered in the film. The acid fast microorganisms are stained pink or bright red whereas the background tissues, cells and other non-acid fast bacilli are stained blue or green.

(iv) Staining of Spores

Bacterial spores are highly resistant to high temperature, radiation, dessication and chemical agents. The ordinary staining dyes do not penetrate the spore walls therefore a specialised technique is used for staining the spores which is described as follows :

(a) As discussed earlier prepare a thin smear on glass slide and heat fix it by passing through bunsen's flame.

(b) Apply the primary stain, malachite green to the heat fixed smear and gently heat to steaming to enhance penetration of the dye into the spores. Continue steaming for about ten minutes. During steaming care must be taken that the stain should not evaporate to dryness.

(c) Wash the slide under running tap water to remove malachite green from cellular parts other than spores.

(d) Counterstain the smear with safranin for 40 seconds.

(e) Wash the slide under running tap water, dry the slide and examine under oil immersion lens. The spores are stained green in colour and vegetative portion of the cell is stained red or pink in colour.

Spore producing bacteria like bacillus anthracia, the causative agent of anthrax and clostridium tetani, the causative agent of tetanus are identified by this technique.

(v) Staining of Capsules

The bacterial capsules are often clearly stained when treated by common stains like crystal violet or methylene blue. The procedure is as follows :

(a) As described earlier prepare a thin film of bacterial culture and air dry.

(b) Stain the slide with 1% crystal violet solution for one minute.

(c) Wash the slide gently with 20% copper sulphate solution to remove excess dye in the capsules.

(d) Examine the slide under oil immersion lens. Staining contrast will be seen between the organism and the capsule. Bacteria is seen as a highly refractile outline against dark background of the dye. The capsular zone is seen as a clear space between the refractile portion and dark background of the dye.

7

COMMUNICABLE DISEASES

Communicable disease is defined as an illness of infectious nature which can spread from one person to another directly or indirectly through an infectious agent or its products from the sick to the healthy persons either by direct contact or through intermediate host, vector, environment (i.e. air, water, soil, dust etc.) or food. Sometimes the infected person does not show the clinical symptoms of the disease and acts as a reservoir of the infectious agent. Such patient is known as carrier. The carrier state can occur in man as well as animal. The carrier state may be short (temporary) or long (chronic).

Certain time period is required for transmitting the infectious agent from diseased person to an healthy person to produce specific disease. This time required is known as communicable period. Depending on the nature of the disease it may be long or short.

Communicable disease is caused when an infectious agent enters the body of an healthy person. The infectious agents which can infect various systems of the body include bacteria, viruses, fungi, protozoa, rickettsia, helminths etc.

With the advancement of civilisation more and more diseases are coming into light and are being investigated. With better knowledge and advancement in their epidemiological studies, these diseases are now being effectively controlled. In developed countries the communicable diseases are practically nil whereas in under-developed and developing countries such diseases are still very common and measures are being taken to control them. Certain communicable diseases are more prevalent in certain areas because of more favourable climatic conditions present over there e.g. communicable diseases are more common in rural and slum areas because of unhygienic conditions which are quite favourable for transmitting the diseases from one person to another person.

For the spread of communicable diseases, three major factors are required i.e.

  (i) Presence of infectious agent e.g. micro-organisms;

 (ii) Presence of susceptible person (host); and

(iii) Favourable environmental factors for its spread.

Unless all the three above mentioned factors are present the spread of disease will not be possible so certain measures should be adopted to control these factors. Certain communicable diseases include chicken pox, measles, influenza, diphtheria, whooping cough, tuberculosis, poliomyelitis, plague, malaria, rabies, syphilis, gonorrhoea, AIDS etc.

A. RESPIRATORY INFECTIONS

Respiratory tract infections are the most common of acute illnesses. The agents for such infections include viruses, bacteria and other micro-organisms. About half of the acute illnesses of upper respiratory tract infections are due to viruses. Inhalation is the commonest route of infection. When a person with respiratory tract infection coughs, sneezes or even talks loudly, fine droplets containing millions of bacteria and viruses are blown into the surrounding air. When these droplets containing bacteria or viruses are inhaled as such or after drying on the floor or clothes by a healthy person may become a source of infection for that person. This kind of infection is known as droplet infection which is the most common way of spreading the diseases. The diseases transmitted by droplet infection include common cold, influenza, measles, whooping cough, diphtheria, chickenpox, tuberculosis etc. Children are more susceptible to such diseases than adults.

1. COMMON COLD

Common cold is a highly communicable disease characterised by inflammation of mucous membrane of nose, pharynx, larynx, trachea, bronchi etc. It is a very common disease and almost everybody suffers from this disease once or twice in a year specially in winter season. Children are more susceptible to this disease. Adults usually recover promptly and completely but viral pneumonia may be fatal to children. If common cold is neglected, it may lead to serious complications of upper respiratory tract. Although during common cold a person may not lie down in the bed but it greatly reduces the efficiency of work. On an average each cold lasts for 1-2 weeks.

Causative Organism

Common cold is caused by a filtrable virus. Any person, if he comes in contact with another person having cold may also get this disease. Other causes of common cold may include sudden changes in temperature, improper food, obstructions of the nose, fatigue, exposure to cold and dampness etc.

Mode of Transmission

It is transmitted by direct contact, by droplet infection or through fomites like handkerchief, towel, book, notebook, pen, pencil etc.

Incubation Period

Incubation period is from few hours to 2-3 days. Sometimes it lasts for seven days. The immunity is short lived.

Signs and Symptoms

During common cold the mucous membrane of the nose becomes swollen and the secretions copious. There is sneezing, running of nose, watery discharge from eyes followed by body ache and head ache. Fever may or may not be present.

Treatment

There is no specific treatment for common cold. Rest is adviseable to give relief from body ache and headache. Analgesics may be helpful in this respect. Common cold generally lasts for a regular course of 1-2 weeks and cures itself, although early treatment shortens the attack. If any body has frequent colds, even though they are not severe, a physician should be consulted because frequent colds may prove harmful to the body.

Prevention

For the prevention of common cold the person suffering from this disease should observe the following precautions :

(i) Preferably he should isolate himself for the first 2-3 days of cold.

(ii) He should keep away from crowded places because coughing and sneezing spread this disease.

(iii) While talking, coughing or sneezing keep a distance from healthy persons and shield the mouth and nose with a handkerchief so that the droplets of infection may not reach to the healthy persons.

(iv) Avoid talking directly into the face of other persons.

2. INFLUENZA

It is an acute highly communicable disease of the upper respiratory tract. In short form it is known as 'Flu'. Influenza tends to spread very rapidly. This is a worldwide infection and causes local or widespread epidemics and pandemics. It affects people of all ages and both sexes and affects millions of persons every year.

Causative Organism

It is caused by a filtrable influenza virus which has three strains namely type A, B & C. Type A causes the most severe type of infection while type C tends to be the mildest.

Mode of Spread

The influenza virus is present in the nasal secretions and the sputum of the patient. The infection is transmitted from one person to another by

(i) direct contact

(ii) droplet infection, and

(iii) through fomites recently contaminated with the virus.

Incubation Period

It is short and varies from 1-2 days. Immunity is also very short which ranges from 6-8 months.

Signs and Symptoms

It is characterised by sudden onset of fever, chill, headache, pain in the limbs and back, sore throat and cough. There is inflammation of the respiratory and gastro-intestinal tract with vomiting. The fever may rise upto 104°F which persists for about 3-4 days. If proper care of the patient is not taken it may lead to some common complications like pneumonia, bronchitis and ear infections which make 'Flu' dangerous.

Treatment

There is no specific treatment for influenza. Antiviral drugs like amantadine or simantidine in a dose of 100 mg twice a day may be given for 3-5 days for the prevention and treatment of influenza.

Prevention

For the prevention of influenza following measures should be adopted:

    (i) Isolate the suspected cases.

   (ii) During illness avoid meeting people for one week.

  (iii) Avoid going to over crowded places.

  (iv) Body should be protected from chills by wearing sufficient warm clothes.

   (v) Face mask should be used while attending a patient.

  (vi) The clothes, beddings, fomites and room used by the patient should be thoroughly disinfected.

 (vii) Sneezing, spitting and coughing in public places should be avoided.

(viii) Saline gargles should be regularly done.

  (ix) Perform regular light exercise, keep fit, take nourishing food, avoid fatigue and chills, and keep in a well ventilated room.

3. MEASLES

It is one of the commonest infectious diseases of children upto six years of age. One attack gives a high degree of immunity even for the whole life. Mother who had an attack of measles imparts immunity to her infants for the first six months of age. This disease has a world-wide distribution. It is endemic but tends to occur in epidemic form every 2-5 years.

Causative Organism

Measles is caused by RNA virus of paramyxovirus group commonly called Rubeola virus. It is present in nasopharyngeal secretions and in blood of infected persons. The measles virus cannot survive outside human body.

Mode of Spread

Measles is one of the most readily transmitted communicable diseases. The mode of spread is direct from person to person, through droplet infection i.e. sneezing, talking, kissing etc. Direct contact with fomite such as spoons, cups and other articles recently contaminated with secretions of nose and throat of the patient may also be a source of transmission of the infection.

Period of communicability is usually 4 days before and 5 days after the appearance of the rash. It is highly infectious during the first few days of illness i.e. during pre-eruptive stage and at the time of eruption of rash stage, afterwards infectivity decreases rapidly.

Incubation Period

Incubation period of measles is 10-14 days.

Signs and Symptoms

Signs and symptoms of the disease can be divided into two stages *viz.*

(a) pre-eruptive stage, and

(b) eruptive stage.

(a) **Pre-eruptive Stage (Prodromal Stage) :** In early stage of the disease or during pre-eruptive stage there is high fever, sneezing, running of nose, watery and red eyes, cough and hoarseness of voice due to laryngitis. Small bluish-white spots on a red base (known as Koplik's spots) can be seen inside the cheeks around the opening of parotid gland. These spots are found in 80 percent cases. The presence of Koplik's spots confirms the diagnosis of the disease. These signs and symptoms last for 3 to 4 days.

(b) **Eruptive Stage :** This stage begins on 4th or 5th day of illness. During this stage a typical dusky-red macular rash appears, first on the face and neck and behind the ears and then rashes rapidly spread all over the body. The rashes are caused by the multiplication of blood borne virus in the skin. The rashes fully appear on whole of the body in about 2-3 days. The rash subsides within 5-7 days leaving a brownish pigmentation of the skin which may last for a long time even after the disappearance of rashes from the body.

Complications

Measles can be a deadly disease particularly in children who are malnourished due to deficiency of proteins, fats and vitamins. Secondary infection may lead to pneumonia, bronchopneumonia, conjunctivitis, stomatitis and gastro-enteritis.

Prevention

The children should be immunised against measles. For this purpose live attenuated, tissue culture freeze dried vaccine is used. A single dose of 0.5 ml of vaccine administered at the age of 9-12 months appears to give 95 percent protection against measles for at least 15 years. It is contraindicated in children who are ill, have history of allergy or are on steroids. When measles vaccine is contraindicated then immunoglobulin can be administered for preventing the infection.

Control

(i) Isolate the patient as soon as the signs and symptoms of measles appear.

(ii) Protect the eyes of the patient from light and glare.

(iii) Disinfect the discharges of nose and throat of the patient.

(iv) Antibiotics may be given to the patient to prevent secondary infection.

(v) Immunise the susceptible children.

4. WHOOPING COUGH (PERTUSSIS)

Whooping cough is a highly infectious disease of the respiratory tract in which trachea, bronchi and bronchioles are involved. It occurs in all ages but more common in children under 5 years of age. It is extremely dangerous if it affects infants under six months of age. Female children are comparatively more affected than male children and deaths are also more common among females.

Causative Organism

Whooping cough is caused by Bordetella pertussis. It is gram negative and is present in nasal and buccal secretions.

Mode of Spread

It spreads directly by droplet infection or indirectly through fomites recently contaminated with patient's nasal and buccal secretions. Children commonly get infection from their playmates who are in early stages of disease. The germs are spread into the air during talking, sneezing or coughing by the patient and when inhaled by the healthy person, gets the disease.

Incubation Period

Incubation period is from 7-14 days.

Signs and Symptoms

There is slight fever, cold, running of nose and irritating cough lasting for a few days to several weeks. During coughing the face becomes red, tears from eyes and vomiting are the common symptoms. At this stage there are severe attacks of irritating cough which becomes paroxysmal producing a typical 'whooping sound' which gives the name to this disease as whooping cough. Paroxysmal attacks of cough are more severe at night.

Infective Period

It is highly infectious during seven days after exposure to three weeks after onset of a typical paroxysm.

Prevention

(i) Every child must be immunised against whooping cough. These days triple vaccine DPT simultaneously gives protection against diphtheria, pertussis and tetanus. Three doses of this vaccine are given intramuscularly at the age of 1½ months, 2½ months and 3½ months. Thereafter a first booster dose is given at the age of 1½ years to 2 years. After this a second booster dose (of DT only) is given at the age of about 5 years.

(ii) Infants should be protected from exposure to this disease.

(iii) The affected children should not be allowed to go to school for a period of six weeks.

Treatment

(i) Isolate the patient.

(ii) Disinfect nasal and buccal discharges of the patient.

(iii) Disinfect the fomites of the patient.

(iv) Cough preparations and antibiotics may be given to the patient.

5. DIPHTHERIA

It is an acute infectious disease affecting most commonly the throat, tonsils, larynx or nose where it produces a greyish white false membrane of a soluble exotoxin. If this membrane spreads to the air passage, it may block entry of air and cause difficulty in breathing. Besides this membrane, the bacteria produce toxin, which if untreated, is absorbed into the blood causing serious complications in the nervous system and heart.

It is widely distributed disease and affects persons of all ages but children in the age of 3-5 years are more affected. Newborn infants are not affected due to immunity received from the mother.

Causative Organism

The disease is caused by the exotoxin produced by corynebacterium diphtheriae. It is a gram positive rod shaped bacteria which grows mainly in the throat, larynx and other portions of the upper respiratory tract. It is found in the secretions of the mouth, nose and throat. It secretes exotoxin which is highly poisonous to man giving rise to toxaemia symptoms. The bacillus is killed by direct exposure to sunlight and heat. It is comparatively a hardy micro-organism.

Mode of Spread

It is spread by droplet infection and through carriers whether sick or healthy. Handling of fomites recently contaminated by nasal or throat secretions also transmit the disease. The droplets containing the bacilli are expelled from the mouth and nose by coughing, sneezing, spitting, speaking or kissing.

Incubation Period

Incubation period varies from 2-5 days but occasionally it may be longer.

Signs and Symptoms

The patient suffers from fever and toxaemia which makes the child miserable. There is difficulty in swallowing and patches of greyish-yellow membrane appear over tonsils and throat. Swabs from this membrane show the presence of the organism.

Prevention and Control

   (i) Efforts should be made for early detection of diphtheria carriers. This can be done by taking swabs from nose and throat and examining for the presence of diphtheria bacilli.

  (ii) Isolate the patient in a well ventilated room.

 (iii) The articles of the patient should be disinfected and good hygienic conditions should be maintained.

 (iv) All infants should be immunised with DPT (triple vaccine) i.e. diphtheria, pertussis and tetanus vaccine starting from the age of 6 weeks. Three doses of DPT are recommended, each consisting of 0.5 ml of vaccine administered intramuscularly at the age of 1½ months, 2½ months and 3½ months. A first booster dose of 0.5 ml of DPT is given at the age of 1½ to 2 years followed by a second booster dose (DT only) of 0.5 ml at the age of 5-6 years. DPT vaccine protects not only against diphtheria but also against pertussis and tetanus.

Schick Test

Schick test is used to find out whether the person is susceptible or immune to diphtheria. This test is carried out by using two diagnostic agents i.e.

   (i) Schick test toxin, and

  (ii) Schick control.

A test dose of 0.2 ml of Schick test toxin is injected intra-cutaneously into the left forearm and an equal volume of Schick control is injected into the right forearm of the individual. The site of each injection is examined on the fourth day. If the left forearm into which toxin has been injected shows redness or inflammation, it indicates that the toxin is not neutralised and the individual is susceptible but if there is no redness or inflammation it indicates that the person is immune. If the redness or inflammation appears it may be due to substances other than toxin which is confirmed from right forearm. If reaction is observed on the right forearm it is confirmed that the person is susceptible to diphtheria but if there is no reaction then the person is immune to diphtheria.

Various types of vaccines used for prophylactic treatment include Alum precipitated toxoid (A.P.T.), Toxin anti-toxin floccules (T.A.F.) and Purified toxoid aluminium phosphate precipitated (P.T.A.P.).

Treatment

(i)   Advise complete bed rest to the patient to prevent cardiac and other complications.

(ii) As soon as the case is detected diphtheria antitoxin must be given immediately in doses ranging from 10,000 to 80,000 units according to the severity of the case.

(iii) Antibiotics like penicillin or erythromycin may be given to eliminate the infection and prevent production of further toxin.

(iv) Fluid diet should be given to the patient till his throat is clear.

(v)   Tracheostomy or laryngeal incubation may be needed if there is respiratory obstruction.

(vi) The household and other contacts may be given a prophylactic dose of 500 to 1000 units of diphtheria antitoxin.

6. CHICKENPOX

Chickenpox also known as varicella is an acute infectious disease. It is a viral infection. Chickenpox occurs mainly in children below 10 years of age but no age however is exempted if there is no previous immunity. One attack generally confers immunity for rest of the life.

Subsequent attacks are rare but in certain cases second attack of chickenpox may also occur.

Causative Organism

Chickenpox is caused by a filtrable virus called varicella zoster virus (V-Z virus) now termed as Human (alpha) herpes virus-3. The virus is so named because it causes both varicella (i.e. chickenpox) and herpes zoster infection.

Mode of Spread

The disease is transmitted from one person to another by droplet infection or by contact with skin. Freshly contaminated articles used by the patient can also transmit the disease.

Incubation Period

Incubation period varies from 14 to 17 days although extremes varying from 7-21 days have been reported.

Signs and Symptoms

There is sudden onset of mild fever and itching. Rash appears in the form of crops on the trunk, face and limbs. Within 24 hours the lesions become pustular i.e. filled with pus. The pustules dry up in a few days to form scabs. Generally chickenpox is mild in children but tends to be more severe in adults.

Prevention and Control

   (i) Isolate the patient.
   (ii) Disinfect all the articles used by the patient.
   (iii) Varicella Zoster immunoglobulin (V-Z 1 gm) given within 72 hours of exposure in a dose of 1.25 to 5 ml by intramuscular injection will impart passive immunity against chickenpox.
   (iv) There is no specific treatment for chickenpox.

7. TUBERCULOSIS

Tuberculosis is a chronic infectious disease caused by tubercle bacilli. It is distributed throughout the world but is more common in developing countries. Three-fourth T.B. cases of the world are found in the developing countries and is an important cause of death is most parts of the world. It is prevalent both in tropical as well as temperate climates and is more prevalent in large over crowded cities and towns. All warm blooded animals are susceptible to this disease and all domestic animals like cow and buffaloes may suffer from tuberculosis which may sometimes be communicated to man.

Tuberculosis is a specific disease which primarily affects lungs and causes pulmonary tuberculosis. It can also affect intestines, meninges of the brain, bones, joints, lymph glands, skin and other tissues of the body. Pulmonary tuberculosis is the most important form of tuberculosis which affects man and will be discussed here.

Tuberculosis can occur at any age but is more common in old persons (particularly males in the age group of 30 year or more) than in young persons. The males are more affected than females. This disease is more likely to occur in persons who are malnourished, who live in over crowded places and where hygienic conditions are poor.

Causative Organism

Tuberculosis is caused by Mycobacterium tuberculosis, an acid fast bacillus discovered by Robert Koch, a German scientist is 1882. Three types of tubercle bacilli are responsible for tuberculosis in man which include human type, bovine type and atypical or anonymous myco-bacteria. The bovine strain affects cattle and other animals.

Mycobacterium is a very hardy micro-organism and can live in dry state for about six months. When exposed to direct sunlight it is killed after eight hours. It is also destroyed by boiling for 10 minutes.

Mode of Spread

(i) It is spread by droplet infection. When the droplets are expelled by tubercular patient through coughing, sneezing, talking and are inhaled by the healthy person.

(ii) By inhaling fine dust particles containing tubercle bacilli derived from dried sputum and other infected discharges thrown on floor, walls, furniture, clothes etc. which after drying get converted into fine particles and mix with dust.

(iii) By handlin sputum and other discharges of the tubercular patient.

   (iv) By direct contact with the patient.

   (v) By consuming articles of food and drinks contaminated with tubercle bacilli.

  (vi) By consuming milk derived from a cow suffering from tuberculosis and without proper boiling.

 (vii) Flies play an important role in transmitting the disease by contaminating the articles of food and drink of healthy persons with tubercle bacilli.

Incubation Period

Incubation period varies from a few months to a few years depending upon the host — parasite contact and severity of infection.

SIGNS AND SYMPTOMS

Early Symptoms

   (i) Excessive fatigue. The patient feels exhausted in an ordinary work. He has general feeling of weakness and does not want to do any work.

  (ii) Slight rise in temperature in the evening.

 (iii) Slight palpitation and rapid pulse.

 (iv) Chest pain.

  (v) Loss of weight.

 (vi) Night sweating.

 (vii) Chronic cough and hoarseness of throat.

(viii) In women, suffering from tuberculosis the mensturation may become scanty or absent.

Later Symptoms

  (i) The body is wasted, cheeks are flushed, eyes sunken and the lips are dry.

 (ii) The breath has peculiar odour and sputum copious (plentiful).

PREVENTION AND CONTROL

General Measures

  (i) One should live in well ventilated house.

 (ii) Streets and buildings should be properly constructed so as to provide plenty of open space.

    (iii) People should be given health education.

    (iv) One should take nourishing and well balanced diet.

    (v) People should be educated not to spit here and there.

    (vi) Milk should be consumed after proper boiling.

    (vii) Unhealthy trades like cotton ginning mills should not be located near the houses where people live. They should be located away from the houses because inhalation of silica and dust particles may lead to tuberculosis.

    (viii) Education and economic conditions of the people should be raised which will lead to overall improvement in standard of living and sanitary conditions.

Specific Measures

    (i) Tuberculosis patients should be detected as early as possible by the examination of sputum, chest X-ray and tuberculin testing. Sputum examination by direct microscopy is now considered the method of choice for early detection of cases and is used all over the world because it is reliable, cheap and easy to perform direct on the sputum.

    (ii) Infected persons should be isolated.

    (iii) All the detected tuberculosis patients should be promptly treated with specific drugs for tuberculosis.

    (iv) The patient shoul not be allowed to spit here and there. He should spit in a sputum cup containing some disinfectant or in a handkerchief which may be cleaned by boiling afterwards.

    (v) While talking or coughing the patient should wear a face mask or keep the handkerchief before his mouth.

    (vi) Patient should be sent to sanitorium.

    (vii) B.C.G. vaccination should be given to newborns below four weeks of age and to the other susceptible cases to protect them against infection. Mass B.C.G. vaccination is done to all individuals below 20 years of age without prior tuberculin test but after 20 years of age B.C.G. vaccination is given only to those persons who are tuberculin negative.

    Bacillus Calmette Guerin (B.C.G.) is named after their discoverers the French bacteriologists Calmette and Guerin. B.C.G. vaccine is prepared from living attenuated bovine strain of tubercle bacilli and freeze dried vaccine is used. It is stored at 4 to 8°C. The vaccine should be used within 4 hours after reconstitution.

Tuberculin or Mantoux Test

This test is performed to find out whether any particular person had any previous tuberculosis infection or not. Sufficient quantity of tuberculin solution (5 tuberculin units) is administered intradermally into the skin of the left forearm. The site of injection is examined after 72 hours (three days). The test is considered positive if there is swelling of at least 6-10 mm in diameter at the site of injection, the redness of the skin is no consideration. Reactions less than 6 mm in diameter are considered negative and B.C.G. vaccination is therefore administered. Preliminary tuberculin testing for newborn infants is unnecessary.

B.C.G. Vaccination

B.C.G. vaccination is usually done to the newborn infants by injecting 0.05 ml of the vaccine intradermally into the skin of the left arm just below the shoulder. In the case of adults the dose of vaccine is 0.1 ml. For injecting the vaccine tuberculin syringe is used. After vaccination there is no general reaction such as fever or pain nor there is any interruption in one's normal work. A local reaction occurs usually 3 to 4 weeks after the vaccination at the site of injection during which a small nodule is formed which heals itself leaving a tiny scar over there. After initial vaccination of the child at birth it is repeated at the age of 5, 10 and 15 years after performing the Mantoux test.

Precautions

    (i) All materials and syringes should be handled aseptically.

    (ii) Both the tuberculin and the vaccine should be stored in a refrigerator.

    (iii) Separate syringes should be used for tuberculin test and B.C.G. vaccination.

    (iv) Always fresh samples of tuberculin and vaccine should be used because they lose their potency after 15 days and seven days storage respectively so the stock must be consumed within this time period and fresh stock recieved from Madras or any other source of supply.

Treatment

Tuberculosis is treated by chemotherapy which includes drugs like streptomycin, isoniazid, PAS (para amino salicylic acid), thiocetazone, viomycin, pyrazinamide, cycloserine, ethambutol, rifampicin etc. The drugs used in the treatment of tuberculosis often develop resistance so single drug is not administered but the patient is put on a combined therapy of two or more drugs at a time and only those drugs should be prescribed which are effective against tubercle bacilli. These drugs should be administered in proper doses regularly and continuously to minimise the risk of drug resistance. The total duration of the treatment is eight months.

B. INTESTINAL INFECTIONS

1. POLIOMYELITIS

Poliomyelitis or infantile paralysis is an acute infectious viral disease of the human alimentary tract but may affect the central nervous system (brain, spinal cord and nerves) resulting in paralysis, the extent of which depends upon the damage done to the nerve cells by the virus. The legs are more affected than arms. If they are only slightly damaged complete recovery is possible but if nerve centre is completely destroyed then the recovery will not be possible leading to permanent disability because the nerve cells once dead cannot grow again. If the nerve cells controlling breathing are affected then the breathing stops and patient dies unless some mechanical device is provided for breathing. It affects all ages but childrein below five years of age are more susceptible. It is one of the main crippling diseases of childhood. It affects both male and female, rich and poor but males are affected more i.e. about three times more than females.

Poliomyelitis is world wide distributed. The developed countries have almost eliminated this disease by widespread use of polio vaccine but polio is most common in developing countries where immunisation against polio is not in wide use. In India a large number of children are affected every year by this disease.

Causative Organism

The causative organism of poliomyelitis is a filtrable virus which has

3 serotypes designated as type 1, type 2 and type 3. Type 1 virus is responsible for most of the outbreaks of polio epidemics.

Mode of Spread

The polio virus is found in the nasopharyngeal secretions, faeces and urine of patients and carriers. Faecal carriers are more dangerous than the nasopharyngeal carriers.

Faecal-oral route is the most common route of transmitting the disease. Infection can spread directly through contaminated fingers or indirectly through contaminated water, milk, food and other articles of daily use. Flies also play a major role in spreading the disease.

Polio may also spread though droplet infection during acute stage of disease when virus is present in pharynx. Close personal contact helps in spreading the disease.

Incubation Period

Incubation period of polio is 7-21 days but may vary from 3 to 35 days.

Signs and Symptoms

In 90 percent cases there are no symptoms, about 8% cases suffer from mild illness and 1-2 percent suffer from major illness when polio virus attacks the CNS and produces varying degree of paralysis.

Pre-paralytic symptoms include high fever, headache, chillness, diarrhoea, vomiting and pain all over the body. Children are drowsy but the adults are restless.

After the pre-paralytic stage there is recovery for 2-3 days and then paralytic stage begins. At this stage pain is produced when an attempt is made to bend the spine forward. The paralysis is of flaccid type and shows great variation in degree and range. The limbs seem to be loose. There is foot drop, facial paralysis and squinting of eyes. If muscles of larynx and pharynx are involved, it may prove fatal sometimes resulting in death of the patient.

Prevention

Polio can be prevented by active immunisation of all infants and children upto five years of age. Oral polio vaccine (OPV) Sabin type is widely used because it is cheap, easy to administer and confers immunity for a long period. It is a live attenuated liquid vaccine. The vaccine is stored at 4°C.

Oral polio vaccine is given in three doses (two drops are put into the mouth as a dose) at the age of 1½ month, 2½ month and 3½ month. One booster dose is given in the same dose at the age of 18 to 24 months. The second booster dose may be given at the age of five years.

Precautions

(i) Polio vaccine should not be given to any child suffering from diarrhoea, dysentery, vomiting and fever.

(ii) Hot milk and hot fluids should not be given to the child at least for half an hour after the administration of the vaccine.

(iii) Vaccine should be stored at sub-zero temperature in a deep freezer to prevent inactivation of the vaccine. For short periods it may be stored in the freezer of the refrigerator. The vaccines prepared now a days are heat stabilized so the problem of storage does not arise.

Other Preventive Measures

(i) The patient should be isolated.

(ii) The faeces, urine and other discharges of the patient should be properly disposed of. The faeces remain infective for 4 weeks.

(iii) Proper provision for safe and adequate water supply and sanitary disposal of solid wastes should be made.

(iv) Hygienic conditions should be maintained.

(v) Flies should be destroyed.

(vi) Avoid over crowding in schools and other places of gatherings.

Treatment

There is no specific treatment for polio. Give complete bed rest to the patient. Antibiotics may be given to prevent respiratory complications. Good nursing care, fomentation and massage help the patient from sufferings. After acute illness, graded physiotherapy helps to a great extent. It helps the weakened muscles to regain strength and become useful again and may prevent crippling.

2. HEPATITIS (VIRAL HEPATITIS)

It is a communicable disease caused by virus and affects liver. The term viral hepatitis includes two major types of hepatitis namely hepatitis A caused by hepatitis A virus (HAV) and hepatitis B caused by hepatitis B virus (HBV).

A. Hepatitis A (Infectious Hepatitis)

Hepatitis A was formerly known as infectious hepatitis. It is distributed throughout the world and usually exists in endemic forms. Children are more affected than adults. An attack of hepatitis A generally provides immunity against a second attack.

Causative Agent

It is caused by hepatitis A virus which is an enterovirus [a virus that enters the body through the gastro-intestinal tract, multiplies there and then (generally) invades the central nervous system]. The virus is found in abundance in the faeces of the patient during early acute phase of the disease and the latter part of the incubation period. Once jaundice develops, it is rarely detectable in faeces. The virus is present in blood for a short period during pre-icteric stage, but usually disappears when jaundice develops. This virus is resistant to heat and chemicals.

Mode of Spread

Hepatitis A spreads by the following modes :

    (i) Faecal–oral route is the major route of transmission. It can occur by using contaminated food, water or milk. Flies may act as mechanical carriers.

   (ii) Disease can spread from person to person by direct contact through contaminated hands or via contaminated articles of use.

  (iii) Transmission of hepatitis A virus is rare through needles, blood or blood products.

  (iv) Infection spreads readily under unhygienic conditions and over crowding.

Incubation Period

Incubation period is 15 to 45 days (usually 28 days).

Signs and Symptoms

It is clinically characterised by fever, chills, headache, fatigue, generalised weakness and pain followed by nausea, vomiting, dark urine, stools are pale coloured, liver enlarged, appetite is lost and jaundice develops. The patient may recover completely in 3 to 6 weeks or in some cases the patient's condition may worsen which may lead to coma and death of the patient.

Prevention and Control

   (i) Isolate the hepatitis cases.

  (ii) Disinfect the faeces and fomites of the patient.

 (iii) Follow personal and community hygienic measures such as washing of hands after toilet and before meals, sanitary disposal of human excreta, using safe drinking water (boiled water should be used during epidemics as virus is not killed by chlorination and by other methods of sterilization) and taking nourishing diet. Enforce sanitary measures in hotels, restaurants and other eating places.

  (iv) Anti-fly measures should be taken.

   (v) Needles and syringes should be properly sterilized. It is advisable to use disposable needles and syringes.

  (vi) Human normal immunoglobulin should be administered to all contacts before or within a week of exposure.

B. Hepatitis B (Serum Hepatitis)

Hepatitis B was formerly known as serum hepatitis. It is an acute systemic infection which affects the liver sometimes leading to cancer of the liver. The disease is endemic throughout the world. It affects all ages but the incidence is more in adults than in children and in urban areas than in rural areas.

Causative Agent

It is caused by hapititis B virus (HBV).

Mode of Spread

   (i) **Parenteral Route** : It is transmitted exclusively by parenteral route through infected blood and blood products, through blood transfusion, dialysis, contaminated needles and syringes, ear or nose piercing, tattooing etc.

(ii) Infection can spread from mother to foetus in uterus.

(iii) Infection may be transmitted by sexual contact or even by kissing.

(iv) Blood sucking arthropods such as mosquitoes and bed bugs can transmit the disease.

The virus is highly infectious and very minute amounts of some carrier serum can transmit the disease. Therefore any method that can convey traces of blood or serum from one person to another can spread the infection.

Incubation Period

Incubation period of Hepatitis B virus is 60 to 180 days.

Signs and Symptoms

The signs and symptoms of hepatitis B are similar to hepatitis A. There is however no history of fever and the onset is more gradual. After the infection there is chronic liver disease which may progress to cancer of the liver.

Prevention and Control

There is no specific treatment for hepatitis B. However the following preventive measures may be helpful :

(i) Avoid blood transfusion and its products which are contaminated with hepatitis B virus.

(ii) Use disposable needles and syringes and always use sterilized instruments for piercing ear or nose or for tattooing.

(iii) Give hepatitis B vaccine by intramuscular route. This vaccine is effective in 95 percent cases and is given in 3 doses of one ml each. The second dose is given one month after the first dose and the third dose is given 5 months after the second dose.

(iv) Hepatitis B immunoglobulin (HBIg) should be given immediately to the persons who are exposed to hepatitis B virus – positive blood e.g. doctors, nurses and attendants engaged in blood transfusion and dialysis work. To be effective HBIg should be given within 24 hours after exposure. It produces passive immunity and provides protection for about three months.

The simultaneous use of hepatitis B vaccine and HBIg is considered superior to the use of HBIg alone.

3. CHOLERA

Cholera is an acute infectious disease of the intestinal tract characterised by sudden onset of severe diarrhoea and vomiting leading to rapid dehydration often resulting in death of the patient. It is both endemic and epidemic disease. It occurs in summer and autumn and generally fades away with the onset of winter. It affects all ages. Mainly people with poor personal and environmental hygiene are affected more. The chances of spread of this disease are more where large number of people get together like fairs, males etc.

Causative Agent

Cholera is caused by two types of vibrios:

(i) Classical cholera vibrios and

(ii) El Tor vibrios.

Mode of Spread

(i) It spreads by ingestion of contaminated water, food, milk, milk products or drinks with discharges of the patient.

(ii) By careless handling of fomites of infected persons and not washing the hands properly thus contaminating the food and drinks themselves.

(iii) Flies act as mechanical carriers.

Incubation Period

Incubation period is very short ranging from a few hours to 5 days (usually 1-2 days).

Signs and Symptoms

Signs and symptoms of cholera include sudden onset of severe diarrhoea (rice water stools) and vomiting. The patient complains of intense thirst, cramps in legs and abdomen. There is suppression of urine followed by rapid dehydration, often resulting in death. Dehydration occurs due to rapid loss of water and salts from the body in stools and vomits.

Prevention and Control

(i) Detect the case as early as possible and immediately notify to the health authorities.

(ii) Isolate the patient in the hospital or at home.

(iii) Give immediate treatment to the patient because minutes and hours count; delay and neglect may prove dangerous.

(iv) During epidemics everybody should be inoculated against cholera.

(v) Patient's clothes and utensils should be thoroughly disinfected.

(vi) Patient's stools and vomits should be collected in a covered pot containing some disinfectant and disposed of immediately.

(vii) All latrines and drains etc. should be cleaned with phenyl or any other disinfectant and sprinkled with lime or bleaching powder.

(viii) Clean and safe drinking water should be used. For drinking purposes water should be consumed after boiling.

(ix) Milk must be boiled before use.

(x) Anti-fly measures should be taken.

(xi) All cut fruits and vegetables exposed to dust and flies should not be eaten, if they are to be used then they must be consumed after thorough washing.

(xii) All foods, drinks and sweetmeats must be protected against flies.

(xiii) It is safe not to use ice, ice cream etc. of doubtful purity.

(xiv) Special care must be taken regarding the cleanliness of the surroundings as well as personal hygiene. One must wash the hands with soap and water after going to toilet and before eating meals.

(xv) Hot drinks and meals should be taken. Taking of curd, lemon juice and butter milk is advisable during epidemic.

Treatment

Each case of cholera can be effectively treated if medical attention is given promptly. The treatment consists of rehydration and antibiotics. During cholera there is great loss of water and salts from the body in diarrhoea and vomiting which leads to dehydration, therefore oral rehydration therapy must be given. For this purpose oral rehydration solution 'ORS' is used, the packets of which are freely available at all dispensaries, primary health centres and other medical centres. Each packet of 'ORS' contains :

Sodium chloride	3.5 gm.
Sodium bicarbonate	2.5 gm.
Potassium chloride	1.5 gm.
Glucose (dextrose)	20.0 gm.

For use, the contents of the packet are dissolved in one litre of safe drinking water and consumed within 24 hours. The solution should be made fresh daily and consumed within 24 hours.

If the above mentioned packet of 'ORS' is not available a simple mixture of common salt (5 gm) and sugar or gur (20 gm) is dissolved in one litre of water and given to the patient.

In severe dehydration intravenous rehydration therapy is given. For this purpose Ringer's lactate solution is used.

Antibiotics are given along with rehydration therapy to cut short the duration of illness. Tetracyline is the drug of choice which is given 500 mg four times a day for 3 days.

4. TYPHOID

Typhoid fever is an acute communicable disease caused by Salmonella typhi. The term 'enteric fever' includes both typhoid and paratyphoid fevers. In the clinical symptoms the paratyphoid fever shows no remarkable difference from typhoid fever.

Typhoid fever occurs in all parts of the world and throughout the year but more in summer and rainy season. The disease affects all ages but more common between 10 to 30 years. It is most common among school going children. An attack of typhoid fever gives a fairly lasting immunity but second attack may also occur.

Causative Organism

Typhoid fever is caused by Salmonella typhi and paratyphoid fever is caused by Salmonella paratyphi A, B or C.

Mode of Spread

Poor sanitation, open air defecation and urination; low standard of living, unhygienic food, contaminated milk and water; illiteracy and health ignorance are responsible for the spread of typhoid fever. Flies also play a significant role in the spread of this disease.

The disease occurs in healthy persons when they take water, milk and food which is contaminated by the stools and urine of the patient or disease can be transmitted directly through contaminated hands or fingers with stools of the patient.

Incubation Period

Incubation period varies from 7 to 28 days (average is 14 days).

Signs and Symptoms

Early symptoms include nausea, vomiting, diarrhoea or constipation, cough, headache, slow pulse rate and fever. In later symptoms i.e. in the second week the fever goes on rising by about one degree every day and reaches to 39.5°C to 40°C which continues for 2-4 weeks. The fever does not come down despite preliminary treatment. The patient feels weakness, tired, there is weight loss, poor appetite and may have pain in the abdomen and enlargement of spleen. If no further complications are involved, recovery begins in the third week. The fever subsides only when specific treatment is given against typhoid or paratyphoid.

Prevention and Control

   (i) Contaminated water is the main mode of spread of this disease so water must be protected from contamination with faeces, urine and sewage. Safe drinking water should be made available to the public.

   (ii) Water and milk should be consumed only after proper boiling.

   (iii) Human excreta and urine which are the major sources of transmission of the disease should be disposed of in a sanitary way.

(iv) Strict sanitation control should be observed in and around the houses.

(v) All eatables should be protected from flies. Raw vegetables and fruits should be washed properly before consuming. Cut fruits and sweetmeats should be covered so as to protect them from dust and flies.

(vi) Antifly measures should be taken.

(vii) Public should be educated for sanitation and personal hygiene.

(viii) All acute cases should be detected, notified and isolated at the earliest.

(ix) Public should be immunised with TAB vaccine which contains S. typhi, S. paratyphi A and S. paratyphi B.

Immunisation is done by injecting subsequently two doses each of 0.5 ml at an interval of 7 to 10 days. Booster doses are required to be given every third year. After injection TAB vaccine causes local reaction, pain, headache, mild fever and swelling.

Treatment

(i) Give complete rest to the patient.

(ii) Give nourishing diet to the patient. Fresh juice of citrus fruits will be quite helpful.

(iii) Chloramphenicol is the drug of choice which should be given by mouth in doses of 500 mg four times a day until the temperature is normal say about 10 days then it is given in doses of 250 mg eight hourly for another 3-4 days to avoid relapse which is very common.

(iv) Stools and urine should be passed in a closed container containing some disinfectant. The container should be cleaned immediately after passing the stools or urine.

(v) All beddings, bed sheets, towels, pillow covers and other articles used by the patient should be thoroughly disinfected and cleaned.

(vi) Great care should be taken for personal hygiene of the patient.

5. FOOD POISONING

Food poisoning is an acute gastro-enteritis caused by ingestion of food or drink contaminated either with bacteria, their toxins, inorganic substances or poisons derived from plants or animals. Food poisoning can occur to a single person or a number of persons at a time. Food poisoning may be classified as follows :

   (a) Chemical food poisoning.
   (b) Food poisoning from plants and animals. In relation to this accidental or delibrate ingestion of poisonous substances that have been mixed with articles of food or drink are not discussed.
   (c) Food poisoning by bacteria and their toxins.

(a) Chemical Food Poisoning

It usually occurs by the use of cheap enamel wares which may contain antimony and if the enamel comes in contact with acidic foods it may dissolve antimony and cause poisoning. Other chemicals which may cause food poisoning include arsenic, cadmium, cyanide, copper sulphate and flourides. Fertilizers, pesticides and adultrants used in agriculture may be another major source of food poisoning.

(b) Food Poisoning from Plants and Animals

Ingestion of certain varieties of poisonous mushrooms may cause food poisoning. Similarly ingestion of certain kinds of fish (Shellfish), meat of infected animals or stale meat may cause food poisoning.

(c) Food Poisoning by Bacteria and their Toxins

Food poisoning by bacteria and their toxins is the commonest cause of food poisoning which is generally caused by ingestion of food and drinks contaminated with bacteria or their products. The bacterial food poisoning is of following types :

   (i) Salmonella food poisoning
   (ii) Staphylococcal food poisoning
   (iii) Botulism

(i) Salmonella Food Poisoning

Salmonella food poisoning is caused by salmonella group of micro-organisms out of which Sal. typhimurium and Sal. enteritidis are the commonest which cause the poisoning. The poison is produced within the body of the bacteria. They are non-sporing and are destroyed by heat but the endotoxins are not killed by heat and can withstand a temperature of 100°C. Foods like milk, milk products, egg, egg products, meat, fish and stored food get contaminated with these bacteria and when ingested, the micro-organisms multiply in the intestine and cause illness in about 12 to 24 hours. The prominent symptoms include acute gastro-intestinal irritation i.e. nausea, vomiting, diarrhoea, pain in the abdomen weight loss, severe dehydration and sometimes death of the patient.

(ii) Staphylococcal Food Poisoning

It is the most common cause of food poisoning. The enterotoxins are produced by staphylococci in foods as a result of the multiplication of bacteria before ingestion. The toxin produced by the bacteria is termed as enterotoxin because of its ability to cause gastroenteritis or inflammation of the lining of the intestinal tract. The organism involved is S. aureus which produces a heat-stable enterotoxin. Due to its heat resistant nature, the toxin cannot be inactivated during normal cooking, and thus causes food poisoning. Staphylococcal food poisoning spreads from ice-creams, milk, milk products, pastries, cakes and when meat in taken in an uncooked or partially cooked form.

The symptoms of food poisoning usually appear 2 to 4 hours after the ingestion of contaminated food which include nausea, vomiting, headache, sweating, and abdominal cramps. In severe cases there is blood and mucous in stools, muscular cramps, a weak pulse and shallow respiration. There may be dehydration due to which patient may die. In severe dysentery and vomiting, a saline solution should be administered intravenously to restore the body fluids and the electrolyte balance.

(iii) Botulism

It is a fatal form of food poisoning which is caused by the ingestion of food contaminated with neurotoxins produced by Clostridium botulinum which is found in under-processed, tinned (preserved) foods, preserved pickles, fruits and vegetables etc. The toxin in produced in preserved foods containing proteins and never in fresh foods. The optimum temperature for the growth of this bacteria and for the production of toxin is considered to be 37°C. The botulinum toxin is thermolabile whereas spores of Clostridium botulinum can withstand storage conditions and remain present in pre-cooked frozen foods. The modern food processing techniques are designed in such a way as to eliminate the heat resistant botulinum spores in food and thus the disease is no longer common now.

The symptoms of botulism appear within 12-20 hours after the consumption of food. The symptoms include nausea, vomiting, diarrhoea headache, dryness of mouth, double vision and decreased salivary secretions. Death may occur in 4-6 days due to heart failure or respiratory failure.

The incidence of bacterial food poisoning is the highest in summer and rainy months due to high temperature and moisture content present in the atmosphere which are quite favourable for bacterial growth.

Prevention and Control

(i) The food animals and meat prepared from them must be thoroughly inspected by a qualified doctor. The food animals and meat should be free from any kind of disease.

(ii) Personal hygiene and food sanitation should be ensured by the individuals particularly engaged in the handling, preparation and cooking of the food. They should be free from infected wounds, boils, diarrhoea, dysentery and other infectious diseases.

(iii) Stored food should be protected from cockroaches, flies, rats, mice and dust.

(iv) Food should be freshly prepared and eaten at the same time. It should be prepared or cooked in clean and good quality utensils so that they do not contaminate the food with chemicals.

(v) Surplus foods should be kept in a refrigerator or cool place because room temperature favours bacterial growth specially in summer season.

(vi) If there is any suspicion that the food or canned food has developed bacterial growth, it must be discarded.

(vii) Strict supervision should be made over resturants, messes or any other place where food is cooked or processed for quality of food and hygienic cooking methods. Food samples must be obtained from these food processing establishments from time to time for laboratory analysis.

Treatment

In case of food poisoning, gastric lavage should be done. When there is severe vomiting and diarrhoea dehydration may occur which should be handled immediately to restore electrolyte and fluid balance by intravenous administration of rehydration solution.

6. HOOKWORM INFECTION (ANCYLOSTOMIASIS)

Hookworm infection is caused by two types of hookworms i.e. Ancylostoma duodenale and Necator americanus. The anterior end of these worms is bent dorsally, hence it is known as hook worm. The male worm is shorter in length than female worm as male worm is about 8 to 10 mm in length and about 0.4 mm thick whereas female worm is about 10-13 mm in length and about 0.6 mm thick. A typical hookworm is almost cylindrical and threadlike with conical head and large oval mouth having four hooklike teeth on the upper side and two knoblike teeth on the lower side of the buccal cavity by which the worm fixes it self to mucous membrane of the intestines.

Mode of Transmission

A single female worm may lay 10,000 to 20,000 eggs per day which are passed in faeces. When they happen to be laid on warm moist soil the eggs hatch into larvae (in about 5 days time) outside the human body in the soil where they grow and develop into infective larvae. They can live in this stage for months when moisture and shade are available, but are rapidly killed by drying. When a person walks bare foot on the contaminated soil, the infective larvae penetrate the skin and enter the body of healthy person. From skin they enter into the blood stream and are carried into the heart and from the heart into the lungs and reach upto trachea and pharynx from where they are swallowed. After swallowing they enter the stomach from where finally they reach the small intestine where they develop into sexually mature worms and start laying eggs in about six weeks.It means an interval of about six weeks is required between the time of initial skin infection and the first appearance of eggs in the faeces. The adult worms attach themselves to the mucous membrane of the small intestines.

Ill-effects of Hookworm Infection

It has been estimated that about 45 million people in India are suffering from hookworm infections. The ill-effects of this disease include iron deficiency anaemia, joint pains, abdominal pain, oedema, general weakness, loss of body resistance and decline in capacity to do hard work.

Prevention and Control

   (i) Defecation in the open should be discouraged because when the moist soil is contaminated with faeces it leads to development of larvae of hookworm.

  (ii) Night soil should be properly disposed of specially in rural and slum areas where chances of spread of this disease are more.

 (iii) Use of sanitary latrines should be promoted in rural areas. This will prevent soil pollution.

  (iv) As a personal protection the peasants working in the fields should wear shoes and gloves for prevention of hookworm infection.

   (v) Habit of walking bare-footed should be avoided.

  (vi) Source of water supply should be protected from contamination with human excreta.

 (vii) Public should be educated for proper use of sanitary latrines as well as personal hygiene specially washing hands after defecation and before taking meals.

In short, hookworm infection can be controlled by adopting sanitary measures, not defecating in the open, proper disposal of human excreta, wearing of shoes and imparting health education to the public.

Treatment

For the treatment of hookworm infection various drugs are available which are quite effective against hookworm. These drugs include mebendazole, albendazole and pyrantal. In areas where hookworm infections are prevalent, community-oriented chemotherapy may be necessary. For the treatment of hookworm anaemia, iron and folic acid should be used and protein rich diet should be given to the patient.

C. ARTHROPOD BORNE INFECTIONS

1. PLAGUE

Plague is highly infectious disease caused by a bacillus bacteria called Yersinia pestis. It is a natural disease of wild rodents and their parasites i.e. fleas because Yersinia pestis is a natural parasite of rodents. Infection is transmitted among them by rat fleas. It is transmitted to man by the bite of infected rat flea present in house rats. Other potential wild carriers are ground squirrels, wood rats and sewer rats.

Mode of Transmission of Plague in Man

The fleas feed on rats and infect them. The infected rats die. After the death of a rat the fleas leave rats in search of food. The healthy rats run away and the starving fleas bite human beings. While biting, the flea regurgitates the plague bacteria from the stomach and thus infects man during the next blood meal causing bubonic plague. The infection may be transmitted by contamination of the bite wound with the faeces of infected fleas. The infection spreads from man to man by droplet infection i.e. during talking, coughing or sneezing.

Types of Plague

In man it occurs in three forms :

    (i) Bubonic plague
    (ii) Pneumonic plague
    (iii) Septicaemic plague

(i) Bubonic Plague

Bubonic plague is the most common form and occurs due to a bite by the infected rat flea. In bubonic plague there is enlargement of lymph glands commonly those in neck, axilla or groins depending on the bite of rat flea i.e. on face, arms or legs respectively. Swelling or enlargement of these lymph glands is known as bubos. Bubones are, however, the most characteristic and important feature of this common form of plague.

Bubonic plague starts usually with a high-grade fever and chill. There may be bodyache, headache and pain in the abdomen as well as diarrhoea and vomiting. The most common feature is the appearance of a 'bubo' which is a painful lymph formed by swollen lymph glands of the neck, groin or axila. It occurs within the first or the second day of illness. It is hard and rubbery to begin with and may become fluctuant later. It eventually breaks down and discharges pus but in mild cases it may resolve without bursting.

(ii) Pneumonic Plague

In this disease the lungs are infected and is transmitted from man to man by droplet infection during breathing, coughing and sneezing by the patient. It is not spread by rat flea. A small proportion of the patients with bubonic plague (about 5 percent) develop pneumonia in the late stage of illness. Such a patient spreads the disease by droplet infection. The onset of the disease is abrupt with shallow breathing and coughing. The sputum is blood stained and contains a large number of bacillus pestis. The disease is uncommon but it is usually fatal.

(iii) Septicaemic Plague

When the organism enters in the blood stream from the infected lymph nodes and infects the whole blood, it is known as septicaemic plague. There may be clotting of small blood vessels in the body. The patient may bleed from multiple sites. In this case the blood infection occurs without the formation of buboes. It is rare and is invariably fatal.

Laboratory Diagnosis

The diagnosis of plague can be confirmed bacteriologically. An aspiration from the lymph node in bubonic cases, the coughed out sputum in pneumonic cases and the blood in septicaemic cases is drawn and examined under the microscope for probable plague bacilli. A bacterial culture is prepared and identified by bacteriological methods.

Incubation Period

It is 3-6 days in bubonic plague but is shorter in pneumonic plague which varies from 1-4 days.

Prevention and Control

Plague can be controlled by the following methods :

(i) Early diagnosis and compulsory notification.

(ii) Isolate the patient and attendants should wear face mask.

(iii) Ensure domestic and community hygiene.

(iv) Garbage must be disposed of at designated places and should not be allowed to pile up.

(v) Keep all food articles covered.

(vi) Adopt anti-rat measures. Houses should be rat proof. Doors and windows should be tight-fitting. All outlets of drains should be covered with a wire mesh. All rat burrows in the house and surroundings should be plugged.

Rats should be trapped or killed with rat poisons.

(vii) Kerosene oil should be put on the dead rats so as to eliminate rat fleas. The carcass should be disposed of in a sanitary method. Rat fleas can also be controlled or destroyed by the spray of DDT and BHC.

(viii) Unusual death of rats should be immediately reported to nearby health authorities.

(ix) Persons with high fever, enlargement of glands, cough with blood in sputum, chest pain and difficulty in breathing should report immediately to nearest health institutions and do not leave the hospital till cured.

(x) Watch out for the above symptoms in persons returning from plague infected areas.

(xi) Do not travel to plague hit areas unless it is absolutely necessary to go there.

(xii) Do not sleep on the floor.

(xiii) Do not panic and do not spread rumours.

(xiv) Do not indulge in self-medication and shun quackery.

(xv) Public should be immunised with plague vaccine.

(xvi) Dead bodies of plague hit persons should be handled with care.

(xvii) Public should be given health education.

Treatment

For the treatment of plague tetracycline is the drug of choice which is given orally in a dose of 500 mg four times a day for 10 days. Sulphonamides are also useful. Wearing of goggles and face masks are also helpful.

WHO experts have pointed out that tetracyclines should not be indiscriminately used. They have warned the public against taking tetracyclines unless they have a risk of exposure to the disease because "every antibiotic has its complications".

2. MALARIA

Malaria is the most important parasitic disease of the world (mainly of the tropical and sub-tropical countries). The term malaria is derived from two Italian words i.e. *mal* means bad and *aria* means air. That means malaria is due to bad air. The incidence of malaria is maximum from April to November. This period is quite favourable for mosquito breeding and female mosquitoes bite human beings for sucking blood. People of all ages and both sexes are susceptible to the infection. There is no natural immunity against malaria. All races are susceptible but Negroes are immune to malaria.

Malaria is the biggest problem in rural areas while in urban areas the mosquitoes are killed by using different kinds of insecticides. In rural areas this problem is more because of insanitary conditions and water remains stagnant at different places including ponds which act as breeding places for mosquitoes, while in urban areas a little care is given to house sanitation and community sanitation. Malaria is such a disease whose appearance may be related to socio-economic status of the society. If one member of the family suffers from fever the other members of the family may also get this disease. Therefore malaria fever must be treated at the earliest. If fever persists for long time it may prove very dangerous and sometimes may lead to death of the patient.

Causative Organism

Malaria is a mosquito-borne febrile disease caused by the malarial parasite (plasmodium) which belongs to class sporozoa. There are four species of malarial parasite which cause malaria in man. These species include :

(i) **Plasmodium vivax :** It has a cycle of 48 hours. Fever recurs after 48 hours or every third day.

(ii) **Plasmodium falciparum :** The fever is very irregular, and may occur every 48 hours. This parasite is responsible for cerebral malaria. It may cause death by attacking the CNS. In this type the attacks are more severe and relapses do not occur.

(iii) **Plasmodium malarae :** It has a cycle of 72 hours. It is a milder form of infection.

(iv) **Plasmodium ovale :** It causes mild fever every 48 hours. It is not found in India but is prevalent in Africa.

In India about 70% cases of malaria are due to P. vivax and 25-30 cases are due to P.falciparum. Malaria cases due to P. Malarae are negligible. All mosquitoes do not spread malaria. It is spread by a particular type of mosquito known as Anopheles that too only by the female anopheles mosquitoes.

Life Cycle of the Malarial Parasite

There are two stages in the life cycle of the malarial parasite first in the man called asexual cycle and the other in the female anopheles mosquito called the sexual cycle.

(i) **Asexual Cycle or Schizogony :** During this cycle the infected female anopheles mosquito bites a healthy person and sucks the blood, at this stage she injects salivary fluid containing sporozoites in the blood circulation. Sporozoites enter the liver where they undergo developmental changes and multiply in the red blood cells of the infected person and give rise to clinical attack of malaria.

(ii) **Sexual or Mosquito Cycle or Sporogony :** This cycle takes 10-14 days to be completed in the female anopheles mosquito. The infective form of the malarial parasite known as sporozoites find their way into the salivary glands from the body cavity of the mosquito and when the female anopheles mosquito bites a healthy person it sucks the blood and injects salivary fluid containing sporozoites in the blood circulation thus causing malaria.

Mode of Spread

(a) Malaria is transmitted by the bite of an infected female anopheles mosquito. During her life time a single mosquito may infect several persons. This type of transmission by the mosquito is known as vector transmission.

(b) Malarial parasite may also be transmitted through infected needles and syringes and by blood transfusion.

Incubation Period

Incubation period varies from species to species. In P. vivax it is 14 days, in P. falciparum it is 12 days. It is the period from the bite of an infected mosquito to the first attack of fever.

Signs and Symptoms

The signs and symptoms of malaria appear in three successive stages :

(a) **Cold Stage :** It is characterised by sudden onset of fever which rises rapidly, headache, bodyache and shivering. This stage lasts for 15 minutes to one hour.

(b) **Hot Stage :** It is characterised by severe headache and very hot flushing of the body and the patient feels like casting off the clothes. This stage lasts for 2 to 6 hours.

(c) **Sweating Stage :** After the last stage there is profuse sweating and temperature becomes normal but the patient feels exhausted. This stage lasts for 2 to 4 hours.

If the infection persists, gradual anaemia develops and the liver and spleen are enlarged.

Prevention and Control

To prevent mosquito breeding and spread of malaria fever following measures should be taken :

(i) Do not allow to collect water around the house and the locality.

(ii) The water meter as well as overhead tanks should not leak or overflow.

(iii) Do not allow to collect the refuse in the dust bins. They should be cleaned regularly and refuse disposed of in a sanitary manner.

(iv) Do not throw the broken earthen pots and other discarded containers/tins/tyres etc. on your roof top because water may collect there which will act as breeding place for mosquitoes.

(v) Do not store water in open containers.

(vi) All water containers, coolers, flowerpots etc. should be emptied once a week, cleaned and dried and then used again.

(vii) All weeds and wild growth should be removed from the locality as well as-banks of small drains and canals so as to eliminate breeding place for mosquitoes.

(viii) All drains should be regularly cleaned and sprayed with D.D.T., B.H.C. or slaked lime.

(ix) Kerosene oil or any other larvicide oil should be sprayed over stagnant water so as to kill mosquito larvae.

(x) Larvicidal fish 'Gambusia fish' should be grown in ponds which will eat mosquito larvae.

(xi) While sleeping in the open, mosquito net should be used.

(xii) Mosquito repellants should be used.

(xiii) Mosquito-proof clothes should be used to prevent bite of mosquitoes.

(xiv) Adult mosquitoes should be destroyed by spraying the insecticides like :

(a) D.D.T. (Dichloro-Diphenyl-Trichloroethane). It is a residual insecticide which is commonly used in the form of emulsion or oily solution for spraying. After the evaporation of the solvent, minute crystals of the insecticide remain on the surface of walls. Mosquitoes have a tendency that after sucking blood they rest on walls and roof of the room, when they rest on these surfaces for some time they absorb some of the D.D.T. through their legs and get themselves poisoned and die after sometime.

(b) 50% D.D.T., kerosene oil solution.

(c) Pyrethrum, D.D.T., kerosene oil mixture (Flit).

(d) B.H.C. (Benzene hexachloride).

(e) Dieldrin.

(xv) Various types of mosquito traps are available in the market which should be used. The mosquitoes are caught in the traps and subsequently killed.

(xvi) Health education should be given to the public.

Treatment

In case of fever it should be assumed that it is malaria fever and presumptive treatment should be given to all such cases. For this purpose 4 tablets each containing 250 mg chloroquin are given to start with. Simultaneously blood slides are prepared and seen under the microscope. If the blood film is positive for the presence of malaria parasite then radical treatment is given which consists of 600 mg chloroquin plus 15 mg primaquin on the first day. Then 15 mg primaquin is given daily for the next four days.

National Malaria Eradication Programme

In India malaria used to be the major killer. Around 1946 100 million persons used to suffer from malaria every year and about 2 million deaths were reported every year. Therefore to control malaria, in 1953, the Govt. of India launched a control programme against malaria known as the National Malaria Control Programme (NMCP) which proved quite successful. Encouraged by the success of the NMCP, in 1958, the Govt. of India switched over to a more ambitious programme known as the National Malaria Eradication Programme (NMEP) with the sole aim of completely eradicating malaria from the country, once for all, in the minimum possible time. A great success has been achieved but in recent years two major difficulties have arisen :

(i) The mosquitoes have developed resistance against DDT, and

(ii) The malarial parasites have developed resistance against drugs.

With the active co-operation of the public to the Government and other societies engaged in this work, the malaria can be totally eradicated from whole of the country.

3. LYMPHATIC FILARIASIS

It is a communicable disease which is transmitted through mosquito bites and exists in acute and chronic forms mainly affecting the . lymphatic system. This disease is not fatal but is a cause of great suffering, deformity and disability.

Lymphatic filariasis is an insect borne disease caused by certain nematodes of the family Filaridae, and is a major public health problem in India. It is found in almost all states of India.

Causative Agent

Lymphatic filariasis is caused by two organisms i.e.

   (i) Wucheresia (Filaria) bancrofti, and

   (ii) Brugia malayi

Out of these two organisms W. bancrofti is more common in causing the infection. They are long thread like tape worms with tapering ends and are easily visible with naked eye. The adult male worms measure about 2.5 cm × 1.0 mm whereas female worms measure about 8 to 10 cm × 0.3 mm in length. Man is the definite host in whose lymphatic system the adult worms live and the culex mosquito is the intermediate host in which the embryos (microfilariae) undergo further development after which they become infective to man.

Mode of Spread

It is spread through bites of infective female culex mosquito. The culex mosquito sucks the blood of an infected person during the night and transmits the disease.

Infection is more common during hot and humid climate which is favourable for mosquito breeding and their development.

Incubation Period

Incubation period is 6-18 months (average 9 months).

Signs and Symptoms

The clinical symptoms are fever, lymphangitis, lymph adenitis, elephantiasis of scrotum, legs and arms due to blockage of lymphatic vessels. Lower extremities are affected more than rest of the parts.

Though this disease is not fatal but it causes great suffering, deformity and disability especially due to swelling of the legs and the external genitalia, a condition termed as elephantiasis.

Prevention and Control

For prevention and control of lymphatic filariasis the measures discussed under malaria for protection from mosquito bite and anti-mosquito measures should be followed.

Treatment

Diethylcarbamazine (DEC) is the drug of choice for treating filariasis. It is available in the market under the name Hetrazan in the form of tablets. Due to its side effects it is not used on mass scale.

D. SURFACE INFECTIONS

1. RABIES (HYDROPHOBIA)

Rabies is an acute and highly fatal viral infectious disease affecting the central nervous system. It is the only comunicable disease of man which is nearly 100 percent fatal. Once the animal gets infected with the disease, he rarely lives more than 10 days.

The term rabies is derived from a Latin word 'rabidus' meaning mad. Rabies is also known as hydrophobia because the patient shows fear from water and is unable to drink water in spite of intense thirst. It is a disease of warm blooded animals like dogs, cats, monkeys, foxes, jackals and wolves. Amongst domestic animals, dog is the commonest source of infection to man. The other domestic animals like cow, horse and camel etc. can be infected when bitten by a rabid dog and hence these animals can transmit the disease to man on biting.

Causative Organism

The causative organism of rabies is lyssa virus type 1 which belongs

to the rhabdovirus group. It is bullet shaped RNA virus. It multiplies
in the nerve cells and is found in saliva, urine, lymph, blood and milk
of infected animals.

Mode of Spread

Rabies is mainly spread by bites of rabid animals (dog is the common
example). It may also spread by licking on a scratched or abraded skin
or mucous of a rabid animal.

Saliva of rabid animals is the most common source of infection.
The rabid dog dies in about 10 days time and its saliva is infective
for first four days. That is why in case of dog bite, the dog in question
is watched at least for a period of 10 days.

Incubation Period

Incubation period varies to a great extent. In man it ranges from 10
days to 8 months or even longer which depends on the site, number
of bites and severity of the bites by the rabid animal. For upper limbs
and trunk it is 40 days, while for lower limbs it is 60 days. It is shorter
in children.

Clinical Features

The disease begins with headache, slight fever, pain at the site of
wound, saliva runs from the mouth. It stimulates all parts of central
nervous system, sensory, motor as well as sympathetic nerves.

The patient cannot tolerate noise and bright light. There is
difficulty in swallowing, fear of water and intense spasms on being
offered food or fluids. The patient dies due to respiratory paralysis or
during convulsions. Once the disease sets in, it is fatal and there is no
treatment of hydrophobia. So its death rate is 100 percent.

Signs and Symptoms in Dogs

When the dog becomes rabid he attacks and bites without provocation,
bites unusual objects such as sticks, straw etc.; runs away from home
and wanders aimlessly biting anything that comes in its way. There
is change in voice and dog barks in a hoarse voice, saliva runs from
mouth in large quantities. The animal dies within 10 days of developing
the signs and symptoms.

Prevention and Control

(i) Clean the wound and scratches with soap and water as early as possible. Then apply spirit or tincture of iodine on the wound and cover it with surgical dressings.

(ii) Observe the biting animal for 10 days, it should not be killed but kept under observation for 10 days. If the animal dies or shows signs of illness within 10 days it means the animal is rabid and antirabies treatment should be started immediately but if the animal survives and shows no signs of illness at the end of 10 days after the bite then the risk of disease is reduced to nil and no antirabies treatment is required except cleaning and dressing of wounds. But antirabies treatment should be given in the following cases :

   (a) When the animal dies or shows signs of rabies within 10 days after the bite.

   (b) When the biting animal has run away and cannot be traced or identified.

   (c) When the bite is from wild animal.

(iii) All stray dogs should be killed and pet dogs should be compulsorily vaccinated.

Antirabies Treatment

The traditional vaccine is the Semple vaccine which is prepared from brain tissue of infected animals. At Kasauli this vaccine is prepared from sheep brain. Vaccine is given subcutaneously in the anterior abdominal wall in a dose ranging from 2 to 5 ml daily for 14 days depending on the severity of the bite.

Now a days cell culture vaccines known as Human Diploid Cell or HDC vaccine have been marketed. It is safe and effective vaccine as compared to Semple vaccine but it is very expensive. This vaccine is given in five doses of 1 ml each by subcutaneous or intramuscular injection (never given at the buttock) at 0, 3, 7, 14 and 30 days and a booster dose is given on 90th day.

2. TRACHOMA

It is a chronic communicable disease of the eye and is an important cause of blindness in the world. More than 15 percent of the world's population suffer from trachoma. In recent years epidemics of conjunctivitis have also been reported.

Trachoma is more common in early summer and monsoon and is related to fly breeding. The children of both sexes are affected more from this disease specially living in unhygienic conditions and overcrowded places. It is also common in school children.

Causative Organism

It is caused by a virus called Chlamydia trachomitis that attacks mucous membrane covering the surface of the eyeball and lining of the eyelids.

Mode of Spread

The disease may spread from one person to another by direct contact or indirect contact, handling of towels, clothes, handkerchiefs, surma or kajal sticks etc. used by infected persons. Swimming pools where water gets contaminated also act as a source of infection. Poor personal hygiene, overcrowding, poverty and malnutrition etc. are the contributory factors to the spread of this disease. Flies also play a major role in spreading trachoma.

Incubation Period

The incubation period varies from 5-12 days.

Signs and Symptoms

In includes development of granular elevations in the conjunctiva (outer covering of the eye), keratoconjunctivitis combined inflammation of the cornea and conjunctiva), epithelial keratitis, pannus, progressive scarring with deformities of the eyelids, secondary bacterial infection and blindness.

Prevention and Control

   (i) Early diagnosis and treatment of the cases should be done.
   (ii) Attempts should be made to remove illiteracy, ignorance, poverty and overcrowding.
   (iii) Health education should be given to parents, children and

students in schools regarding the spread, prevention and control of trachoma.

(iv) Common use of eye preparations, towel, handkerchief etc. should be avoided.

(v) Defecation in the open should be discouraged.

(vi) Anti-fly measures should be taken.

Treatment

Treatment of trachoma consists of giving tetracyclines and sulpha drugs for oral administration and 1% tetracycline eye ointment is applied daily twice a day. Deformity of eyelids require surgical treatment. Proper attention should be paid to personal hygiene.

3. TETANUS

Tetanus or lock jaw is an acute disease which is distributed throughout the world. Being associated with socio-economic and hygienic conditions, the incidence is higher in developing countries. It occurs throughout the year but hot damp climate is favourable for the development of spores. It is more prevalent in rural areas than in urban areas.

Neonatal tetanus is a major cause of infant mortality in India. Many mothers also die after child birth because of tetanus caused by unsafe delivery practices. These deaths may be due to improper and unhygienic cutting of umbilical cord after birth with dirty and rusted blades. Sometimes unhygienic dressings used may also cause tetanus. Neonatal tetanus can be prevented by giving every pregnant woman two doses of tetanus toxoid and maintaining sterile conditions during child birth.

Causative Organism

Tetanus is caused by the exotoxin produced by Clostridium tetani. It is a gram positive spore bearing bacteria which is present in the faeces of man and animal. The spores germinate under anaerobic conditions and produce a powerful exotoxin.

Mode of Spread

It is always through injury and abrasion from where the contaminated matter with tetanus spores enter into the body. The road side injuries and injuries caused by iron articles are the major causes of tetanus. The other causes of tetanus include pin prick, abrasion, wound, burns, human bite, animal bite, stings, use of unsterile injectable needles and syringes as well as surgical instruments. Tetanus may also be caused when spores are introduced through surgical catgut, dressings and various powders such as talcum and sulphonamides etc.

Incubation Period

Incubation period varies from 3 to 21 days.

Signs and Symptoms

The first symptoms of tetanus usually appear from 3 days to 3 weeks, after the micro-organisms enter the body through the wound. The first indications of the trouble are irritability, restlessness, headache, and fever. Gradually the neck becomes stiff and there is difficulty in chewing and swallowing. Subsequently spasms of muscles of the jaw and face take place and thus 'Lock jaw' occurs. The temperature may rise even upto 105°F. There is severe pain and a large number of patients die after a few days. Mortality rate tends to be high varying from 40 to 80 percent.

Prevention and Control

(i) Tetanus can be prevented by giving active immunisation with tetanus toxoid. It is the most effective, safest and practical method of tetanus prevention.

(ii) Infants and children are best immunised by giving DPT i.e. diphtheria, pertusis and tetanus triple vaccine. Every child should be vaccinated with DPT vaccine. Three doses of 0.5 ml at one month interval are given followed by another dose after a year or so. Thereafter booster doses of 5-10 years intervals are given to maintain immunity.

(iii) Pregnant women should be given tetanus toxoid doses as a routine to prevent neonatal tetanus.

(iv) Complete sterility precautions should be taken during child birth.

(v) All wounds should be thoroughly cleaned and long acting penicillin (benzyl penicillin) should be administered. It strongly inhibits the growth of Clostridium tetani and stops further production of toxin.

(vi) The patient should be given muscle relaxants and sedatives. He should be kept in a dark and calm room free from noise.

(vii) The patient with a wound should be immediately given an injection of ATS or human tetanus immunoglobulin. This is the best prophylactic measure against tetanus and provides passive immunity to the patient.

ATS has certain disadvantages that it is rapidly excreted from the body and causes sensitivity reactions in certain persons therefore the use of ATS is discontinued in many countries and in its place human tetanus immunoglobulin is used.

4. LEPROSY (HANSEN'S DISEASE)

Leprosy is a chronic, communicable disease, being curable and non-hereditary. It is distributed throughout the world. In India there are about 1/3rd of world's total of leprosy cases. All ages are prone to infection although children are affected more. Male are more affected than females. The disease mainly affects the skin, peripheral nerves, muscles, bones, eyes, testes, nasal mucosa and internal organs.

Classification

Leprosy is classified in two varieties :

(i) **Non-infective :** It is generally known as Neural or "Non-Lepromatous". It is further classified into two sub-groups i.e.

(a) leprosy with patches on the skin, and

(b) leprosy without patches on the skin.

(ii) **Infective :** It is known as 'lepromatous leprosy'. The patient suffering from infective leprosy sheds germs from the nose, throat and skin.

Causative Organism

Leprosy is caused by Mycobacterium leprae which is an acid fast bacillus. It was first discovered by a leprologist of Norway named Armaur Hansen in the year 1675. That is why this disease is also known as Hansen's disease after his name.

Mode of Spread

Leprosy is transmitted through (a) prolonged skin contact with infected person either directly (skin to skin) or indirectly through fomites; (b) droplet infection when the bacilli escape from the cutaneous lessions, nasal and sputum secretions. The bacilli can also be transmitted to the infants through mother's milk suffering from leprosy.

Incubation Period

Incubation period is long and varies from a few months to a number of years. Commonly it varies from 6 months to 8 years.

Signs and Symptoms

In the first stage initially there is an appearance of a small patch on the skin. It has less sensation than the surrounding area of the skin.

In the second stage the skin of the face becomes thick and wrinkled, ears are swollen. Nasal and throat discharges contain lepra bacilli which are even passed in urine and faeces. This stage is highly infectious.

In the third stage the discharges contain very few lepra bacilli and the patient is less infectious. During this stage certain deformities of hands and feet take place. The fingers and toes become bent, ulcerated or drop and disappear altogether. The patient is thus progressively disfigured and crippled.

Prevention and Control

(i) Cases of leprosy should be notified.

(ii) Lepromatous patients should be isolated in their homes, hospitals or institutions.

(iii) Infants should be separated at birth from lepromatous parents.

(iv) Lepers should not be allowed to roam in the streets or bazars.

(v) Their discharges, clothes etc. should be destroyed or thoroughly disinfected.

(vi) Pepole should be given health education.

(vii) Leprosy should be treated with multi-drug therapy. A combination of rifampicin, dapsone and clofazimine is recommended. DDS (diamino diphenyl sulphone) is marketed as dapsone. Use of penicillin and streptomycin is also helpful for the control of secondary infections.

E. SEXUALLY TRANSMITTED DISEASES (STD)

These are a group of communicable diseases which are transmitted by sexual intercourse and are caused by a wide range of bacterial, viral, protozoal and fungal agents and ectoparasites. Formerly the sexually transmitted diseases were known as venereal diseases and are one of the acute public health problems. Many instances of broken homes, family unhappiness and high infant mortality rate can be attributed to sexually transmitted diseases which may be due to marital disharmony, poverty, alcoholism and family quarrels.

The basic social factors responsible for the spread of sexually transmitted diseases is prostitution which is quite high in large cities, ports and pilgrim centres, where there are more men and less women and where men are forced by circumstances to remain separated from their families. Modern publicity in books, nude films, television and advertising lead the young boys and girls to indulge in undesired sexual practices. Moreover lack of discipline in the family and parental supervision contributes to the worsening of the situation. Urbanisation is another major factor responsible for this problem. STD are more prevalent in the 20-40 years age group. The examples of STD include syphilis, gonorrhoea, chancroid, lymphogranuloma venereum (LGV), AIDS etc.

1. SYPHILIS

Syphilis is a chronic infectious disease which occurs throughout the world but in western countries its incidence has been decreased to a great extent due to strict laws and better medical facilities.

The disease is self-inflicted because wounds remain hidden and unnoticed due to stigma and shame. Untold sufferings of a large number of people goes unnoticed and the disease continues to spread in spite of the availability of specific treatment.

Causative Organism

Syphilis is caused by Treponema pallidum. It is a spiral shaped germ which has 8-15 spirals which passes through cracks in the skin or mucous membrane.

Types of Syphilis

Syphilis is of two types :
  (a) Acquired syphilis
  (b) Congenital syphilis

(a) Acquired Syphilis

Generally adults and elderly persons get this disease through sexual intercourse whereas children get this disease through kissing or fondling of sex organs. The patient of syphilis passes through three stages :

  (i) **Early Syphilis or Primary Stage :** During this stage a hard sore called chancer appears on genitals in 2-6 weeks time. This sore is hard, almost painless, without itching and there is no discharge. It heals up itself leaving behind a scar.

 (ii) **Secondary Stage :** This stage appears 6 weeks to 6 months after the infection. During this stage there is enlargement of glands, headache, sore throat, and low irregular fever. Loss of voice and loss of hair are also seen.

(iii) **Tertiary Stage :** This stage may appear after 5 years of infection. It affects almost all organs of the body. During this stage lesions appear almost anywhere but the skin, bones, tongue, testes, liver, heart and CNS are affected more. Gumma, a chronic granulomatous lesion of the internal organs appears which is not painful and tender.

(b) Congenital Syphilis

Congenital syphilis occurs from birth because the infection is passed from the mother to the faetus through placenta. In congenital syphilis mother does not conceive, if pregnancy occurs after repeated abortions there may be still birth of 2 or 3 children in 3rd, 6th and 7th months of pregnancy respectively. If third or fourth child is born alive he may be a defective child both physically and mentally.

Mode of Spread

The acquired syphilis is spread through sexual intercourse whereas the congenital syphilis is transmitted from the infected mother to the child through placenta. Syphilis may also spread through infected towels, kissing and .fondling of sex organs.

Incubation Period

Incubation period varies from 10 days to 10 weeks. Average is 3 weeks.

Treatment

Procaine penicillin is the drug of choice which can be given in early stages in a daily dose of 6,00,000 units intramuscularly for 10 days. For secondary syphilis it is given in double dose for 20 days. In tertiary syphilis the course of procaine penicillin is repeated several times.

2. GONORRHOEA

It is an acute infectious venereal disease. It occurs in two stages.

(i) **Acute Stage** : This stage is characterised by inflammation of urethra in males. Sometimes it also occurs on the cervix and vagina of females. There is an acute burning sensation with pain and pus discharge while passing the urine. Later the pus becomes thin and perists for a long time. In males the infection spreads to the prostate gland, seminal vessicle and urinary bladder. In females it spreads to the uterus, peritoneum and bartholin glands. Females spread the disease more because they do not suffer much pain and infection remains hidden in the cervix. Later on the infection spreads to heart muscles, joints, eyes and meninges of brain through blood.

(ii) **Chronic Stage** : In this stage the stricture of urethra occurs followed by inflammation of big joints like shoulder joint, knee joint, wrist and ankle. The females may become sterile when infection spreads through fallopian tube.

Causative Organism

It is caused by Neisseria gonococcus which is a gram negative diplococcus. It is a very sensitive organism and is easily destroyed by drying and even with weak disinfectants.

Mode of Spread

Gonorrhoea is transmitted through sexual intercourse with an infected partner. In certain cases it may spread indirectly through infected towels, bed sheets, clothes etc. but it is rare since the germs die readily outside the body.

Incubation Period

Incubation period varies from 3 to 10 days.

Treatment

Procaine penicillin is the drug of choice which is given 6,00,000 units intramuscularly as a single dose. The other drugs which can be given include benzyl penicillin sodium plus probenecid; ampicillin with probenecid; and septran.

Prevention and Control of Sexually Transmitted Diseases (STD)

STD can be prevented by adopting following measures :

   (i) All cases of STD are generally associated with some other case hidden in the family or in the community. So that case must be found out which will help in controlling STD.

 (ii) There is a tendency among STD cases that they discontinue the treatment before the disease is controlled so effective and complete treatment should be given to the patients.

(iii) Condom should be used during intercourse.

(iv) Prostitutes should be licensed and they should be medically examined from time to time for the absence of STD.

 (v) Prostitution, broken homes, family quarrels, marital disharmony, poverty and alcoholism etc. which are the root causes of STD, should be tackled properly so as to overcome these problems and rehabilitate them.

(vi) Overall living conditions should be improved.

(vii) Impart health education to the public because it is an important component of STD control programme. They should be educated about the problem of STD in the community and they should be motivated to adopt some suitable measures to overcome this problem for themselves and for the community.

3. AIDS

AIDS stands for Acquired Immuno Deficiency Syndrome which is a very fatal disease. This disease is caused by a virus known as human immunodeficiency virus (HIV). HIV attacks the white blood cells which serve as the body's defence system against infections. Once these cells are infected with HIV, this defence system gets weakened, exposing the body increasingly to infections that ultimately prove fatal.

Since the AIDS virus reduces the natural immunity of the human body therefore persons suffering from AIDS become easy target to many other infections or diseases. The persons suffering from AIDS actually die from other infections or diseases which attack the body due to weakend state of immunity. This is because the human body cannot resist the disease causing organisms under those conditions when its natural defence mechanism has been destroyed by AIDS virus. AIDS is incurable hence invariably fatal. At present there is no vaccine available against HIV infection.

Causative Organism

AIDS is caused by a virus known as human immunodeficiency virus (HIV).

Mode of Spread

HIV virus is transmitted from one person to another by following methods :

(i) Sexual contact i.e. vaginal, oral or anal sex can spread AIDS as the virus is excreted in the semen or vaginal secretions.

(ii) Through transfusion of blood infected with AIDS virus.

(iii) Through contaminated needles and syringes.

(iv) It is transmitted from infected mother to the foetus through placenta.

A person suffering from other sexually transmitted disease runs a very high risk of acquiring the AIDS virus because STDs usually, cause ulcers, sores or discharge, the HIV enters more easily through these openings in the skin.

The following persons are most exposed to AIDS :

(i) People with multiple sexual partners.

(ii) Truck drivers and others visiting prostitutes.

(iii) Persons getting limbs tattooed/ears pierced.

AIDS does not Spread

(i) Through shaking hands.

(ii) Through causal social contact with the patient.

(iii) By playing with infected person.

(iv) By sharing food, towels, clothes and toilets.

(v) Through mosquito or other insect bites.

Incubation Period

Incubation period is 10 years.

Signs and Symptoms

Signs and symptoms of AIDS include

(i) Weight loss.

(ii) Fever or night sweating for longer than one month (intermittent constant).

(iii) Chronic diarrhoea which persists for more than one month.

(iv) Swelling in the groins.

(v) Purple spots on the skin.

(vi) Persistent cough and shortness of breath.

Prevention and Control

At present there is no vaccine or cure for treatment of HIV infection or AIDS. Until a vaccine or cure for AIDS is found the best is to adopt suitable measures by which AIDS can be prevented. The following preventive measures should be adopted :

(i) Have only one uninfected sexual partner and do not indulge in multiple sexual partners.

(ii) Avoid going to prostitutes for sexual intercourse.

(iii) Do not indulge in oral/anal sex.

(iv) Use condom during sexual intercourse.

(v) Properly sterilise the needles and syringes. Preferably use disposable needles and syringes.

(vi) Women suffering from AIDS or who are at high risk of

infection should avoid becoming pregnant because infection can be transmitted from infected mother to unborn or newly born child.

(vii) Blood and blood products should be thoroughly investigated for the absence of HIV infection.

(viii) Avoid blood donation from strangers and professional donors.

(ix) Hair cutting saloons should ensure that barber's razor is properly cleaned.

(x) Piercing of nose, ear lobes or tattooing carry a risk of HIV transmission therefore instruments used for this purpose should be thoroughly sterilized.

(xi) Impart health education to the public to enable them to make life-saving choices (e.g. avoiding indiscriminate sex, using condom etc.).

AIDS is quite common in western countries because of the undesirable sexual practices, polygamy and polyandry. In India also AIDS is increasing at an alarming rate. The most unfortunate part is that no medicine or vaccine has been developed so far which can prevent or cure AIDS. Therefore once a person gets AIDS he is sure to die in a short span of life that is why it is labelled as 'AIDS the other name of Death'.

8

NON-COMMUNICABLE DISEASES

A non-communicable disease is a disease which is not transmitted directly or indirectly from one person to another but it is caused due to multiple causes. In developing countries, communicable diseases constitute one of the most important problems but in the developed countries, non-communicable diseases have become the leading problem. Such diseases include cancer, diabetes, cardio-vascular diseases, blindness, obesity, accidents and various other metabolic and degenerative diseases.

The pattern of disease problem in a country changes with ways of living as well as with the health care programmes. Epidemiological studies of these diseases and problems aim at finding out nature and extent, causes, diagnosis, prevention and control of these problems. The causes are mostly social, cultural, psychological, mental and environmental. With fast urbanization and industrialization the stress and strain in life is increasing which has led to rise in non-communicable diseases. It is more difficult to control non-communicable diseases than communicable diseases because the cause of the disease may lie in the life-style which is difficult to change e.g. smoking is the cause of lung cancer and asthma. In diabetes and hypertension genetic factors play important roles. Due to these reasons non-communicable diseases are difficult to treat. However preventive measures help to a great extent in controlling the non-communicable diseases.

Risk Factors for Non-Communicable Diseases

The following factors are considered responsible for majority of non-communicable diseases :

- (i) Smoking or chewing of tobacco.
- (ii) Drinking of alcohol.
- (iii) Customs, habits and life styles.
- (iv) Environmental factors i.e. air, water, light.
- (v) Inadequate health services for management and control of non-communicable diseases.

1. CANCER

Cancer is one of the major causes of deaths all over the world where communicable diseases have been controlled. Cancer can occur in any part or any tissue of the body and can involve any type of body cells. Common types of cancer are oral cancer, oesophageal cancer, cancer of cervix uteri, lung cancer, stomach cancer, gall bladder cancer, hepatic cancer, breast cancer etc. Oral and oesophageal cancers are among the most malignant diseases in India, mostly due to habit of smoking and tobacco chewing. Cancer of cervix uteri and breast cancer are very common in females but these types of cancer are relatively rare in unmarried women.

Penile cancer is common is men which is due to accumulation of smegma under the prepuce. If hygienic measures for penile cleanliness are adopted then such type of cancers can be reduced to a great extent.

Causes of Cancer

Cancer is caused due to

- (i) An abnormal and purposeless multiplication of cells in size and mass more than they should.
- (ii) The ability to infiltrate to the adjacent tissues or distant organs.
- (iii) Because cells are not dying when they should.
- (iv) If the tumour has developed to such an extent that it can't be removed successfully then ultimately death of the patient will be the result.

Contributory Factors for Causes of Cancer

The following agents are the contributory factors for causes of cancer:

(i) Chemical agents e.g. coal tar dyes and its derivatives, soot, aromatic amines, benzedine, asbestos, nickel etc.

(ii) Physical agents e.g. X-rays, ultraviolet rays and radiations.

(iii) Mechanical agents e.g. friction, trauma and irritation.

(iv) Biological agents e.g. virus is supposed to be involved in cancer causation and factors like schistosomiasis in urinary bladder cancer.

Along with the above mentioned factors other contributory factors for causation of cancer include age, sex, occupation, marital status, socio-economic status, heredity, environmental factors, and customs and habits. Chances of development are more with the advancement of age. Breast cancer and cancer of cervix uteri is more in women specially married one. Persons who are in the occupation of dealing with chemicals such as benzene, arsenic, cadmium, chromium etc. are exposed to development of cancer. Customs and habits like consumption of alcohol, smoking, chewing of tobacco or paan, use of hot spicy food etc. all contribute to the causation of cancer of one organ or the other.

Signs and Symptoms

The following are the danger signs of cancer :

(i) Any sore that does not heal.

(ii) Formation of lump, tumour or thickening in the breast or else-where in the body.

(iii) Unusual bleeding or discharges from any part of the body.

(iv) Difficulty in swallowing and persistent indigestion.

(v) Persistent cough or hoarseness of voice.

(vi) Any sudden changes in skin and outgrowth of skin like wart and mole.

Prevention and Control

Cancer can be prevented if following measures are adopted :

(i) Try to avoid consumption of alcohol and tobacco in any form.

(ii) Try to avoid and protect against known carcinogenic agents such as chemicals, drugs and radiations.

(iii) Ensure personal hygiene to prevent the cervix and penile cancer.

(iv) Persons should be immunised against hepatitis B virus to prevent liver cancer.

(v) Food, drugs and cosmetics should be tested for their carcinogenic activity.

(vi) Early detection and treatment of precancerous lesions should be done. For this purpose cancer detection centres should be established.

(vii) Breast cancer should be detected at an early stage through mammography and steps taken to control breast cancer.

Millions of women today suffer from this deadly disease. Moreover the number of such cases are increasing day-by-day. The changing life style correlates with delayed child bearing (after 30) the early onset of menstruation (before 12) and late menopause (after 50) are the risk factors for breast cancer.

(viii) Mass surveys and screening should be done especially in old people.

(ix) After cure, rehabilitation of cancerous patients should be kept in view.

Treatment

For the treatment of cancer surgery, radiotherapy, chemotherapy and immunotherapy are needed. Now-a-days instead of giving one therapy a combination of two or more than two therapies are given to control cancer and this has become the general practice in cancer centres all over the world. The latest technique for treating cancer is the laser therapy i.e. Interstitial Laser Photocoagulation in short form known as ILP.

The patients who cannot be treated by above mentioned therapies and have crossed the curable stage, they must be provided with some pain killers so as to give relief from unbearable pain.

2. DIABETES MELLITUS

Diabetes mellitus (D.M.) is a disorder of glucose metabolism which is either due to

(a) Inability of pancreas to produce sufficient insulin needed for the body, or

(b) Inability of the body cells to use the insulin available.

The normal blood glucose level ranges from 70-90 mg per 100 ml but if the fasting blood sugar level increases more than 120 mg per 100 ml then diabetes mellitus should be suspected. If the blood sugar is more than the normal concentrations then it is known as hyperglycemia but when the blood sugar level is less than the normal concentration then it is known as hypoglycemia. Hyperglycemia is characterised by high concentration of sugar in blood and the presence of sugar in the urine (glycosuria).

Diabetes mellitus is a disease that occurs throughout the world and about 30 million diabetics are there in the world. The incidence of diabetes is increasing because female diabetics are able to have children. The incidence of diabetes is higher in persons above 40 years of age. Females especially the married ones are more prone to get this disease. Obesity, dietary factors and heredity are the other contributory factors for diabetes. Alcoholic beverages increase appetite, encourage weight gain and when taken in excess damage the pancreas and thereby increase the risk of diabetes.

Diabetes could be caused not only by deficiency of insulin but also due to disturbances in the level of certain other substances like adrenaline, pitutary hormones, thyroid hormones, oestrogens, corticosteroids, glucagon etc. All these substances produce their effect on blood sugar level so glucose tolerance curve should be determined which will be most useful test for diabetes.

Types of Diabetes

Clinically diabetes is of two types :

(i) **The juvenile onset type or insulin dependent diabetes (IDDM):** This type of diabetes usually develops at a young age during first 40 years of life and has a very rapid onset. In this type of diabetes the pancreas produces very little or no insulin so administration of insulin is required hence it is called insulin dependent diabetes.

(ii) **The adult or maturity onset type or non-insulin dependent diabetes (NIDDM) :** This type of diabetes usually develops after

40 years of age or elderly persons who are obese and progresses slowly. In this type of diabetes, the pancreas produces inadequate amount of insulin. This type of diabetes can be controlled by dietary control alone and light exercise or along with oral hypoglycemic drugs.

Signs and Symptoms

   (i) Frequent urination and passing large volume of urine.

  (ii) Increased thirst.

 (iii) Increased appetite.

  (iv) Loss of weight.

   (v) General weakness and fatigue.

  (vi) Pain in the legs.

 (vii) Irritability.

(viii) Lack of concentration.

  (ix) Prone to infection.

   (x) Delayed wound healing.

All diabetics do not have all these symptoms but from No. (iv) to (x) are definite indications of diabetes.

Possible Complications of Diabetes

Slow blood circulation in legs, heart disease, kidney failure, poor vision, numbness, parasthesia, feeling of pins and needles, loss of sensation are some of the common complications of diabetes but if the blood sugar is controlled to normal range i.e. 120-150 mg per 100 ml then most of the above mentioned complications can be prevented.

As a result of long-term complications like heart disease, kidney damage and even blindness may occur. As compared to a non-diabetic, the risk of diabetic getting a heart attack is two times more, four times for gangrene, 17 times for kidney failure and 25 times for blindness.

Prevention and Control

Diabetes cannot be cured but can be effectively controlled so that a diabetic can enjoy life, feel hale and hearty. Life expectancy in a well controlled diabetic is the same as that in a non-diabetic. Diabetes can be prevented and controlled by adopting following measures :

(i) The diabetic case should be detected as early as possible. A prediabetic has no symptoms of diabetes, has normal blood sugar but shows impaired glucose tolerance curve.

(ii) A diabetic should not marry to another diabetic otherwise their children will also be diabetic.

(iii) The obesity should be reduced by restricting the diet and going for normal physical exercise.

(iv) The body weight should be 10 percent less than the normal body weight.

(v) Personal hygiene including care of feet and skin should be taken care of.

(vi) Regular check up of urine sugar and blood sugar should be done.

(vii) The patient should try to avoid emotional and social stress and strain in life which are associated with diabetes.

Treatment

Diet, physical exercise and drugs are recommended for treatment of diabetes. The treatment should be done under the supervision of a qualified diabetologist and supervised by him once in three months. The patient should undergo full biochemical tests, eye check up and obtain advice for foot care at least once a year. The commonly used drugs in controlling the diabetes are insulin which is administered by parenteral route in case of insulin dependent diabetes. For non-insulin dependent diabetes various types of oral tablets are available. These tablets belong to a class of compounds known as sulphonylurea. These tablets include Daonil, Diabenese, Glynase, Ratinon, Euglucon etc. These tablets are better absorbed from empty stomach so they should be taken 15-30 minutes before meals once or twice a day or as suggested by the physician.

Diabetes is a disease which leads to many complications such as blindness, kidney failure, coronary thrombosis and gangrene of lower limbs therefore blood sugar level must be maintained between 80-150 mg per 100 ml to prevent majority of the complications that arise from diabetes. For this purpose he must get the expert advice from a qualified diabetologist by getting himself registered with specialised clinics known as diabetic clinics for the diagnosis and treatment of diabetes.

3. BLINDNESS

A person is considered blind if his vision is less than 1/20th of normal vision or if he is unable to count fingers at a distance of 1½ metres. In India nearly 12 million blind people exist and the number is gradually increasing due to industrialisation, malnutrition, poverty and so many other factors discussed below.

Causes of Blindness

   (i) Communicable diseases responsible for blindness are smallpox, measles, leprosy, trachoma and sexually transmitted diseases.

  (ii) Non-communicable diseases responsible for blindness are diabetes, hypertension, diseases of the nervous system, tumour of the eye, cataract and associated infections of the eye, retinal detachment, glaucoma and injuries of the eye.

 (iii) Malnutrition specially vitamin A deficiency is also an important cause of blindness.

 (iv) Faulty posture, glare, poor lighting and refractory errors also cause blindness or defective vision.

  (v) Occupation of the persons is also important factor for blindness. Persons working in industries, mines etc. get injury of the eye very often.

 (vi) Poverty, illiteracy, inadequate health services and poor sanitation may also cause blindness.

(vii) Superstition and treatment by quacks may also lead to blindness.

Prevention and Control

   (i) Any discharge, redness or pain in the eye should be taken note of seriously and immediate measures should be taken to find out the cause and treated properly.

  (ii) Eye diseases like conjunctivitis, ophthalmia neonatorum, superficial foreign bodies etc. should be treated at the earliest by a trained person.

 (iii) Common blindness causing diseases like cataract, eye trauma, glaucoma etc. should be treated by organising camps in villages or in the hospitals.

   (iv) Health education and personal hygiene regarding eye care should be given to the public.

   (v) Occasional doses of concentrated vitamin A to children are helpful in preventing blindness.

  (vi) Special schools for the blind for their proper training and rehabilitation should be started so as to lessen the unproductive expenses on the blind and turn them into productive ones. They should be trained in such a way so as to give them gainful employment.

Specific Programmes for Prevention of Blindness

A national programme for the prevention and control of blindness was started by the Govt. in the year 1976. According to this programme the target is to reduce the incidence of blindness to 0-3 percent by 2000 A.D. To achieve this target following programmes are undertaken :

   (i) Eye check up of children is done in schools.

   (ii) Vitamin A prophylaxis is done by giving vitamin A solution orally to all children upto six years of age.

  (iii) Eye camps and permanent eye care facilities are established.

  (iv) More and more ophthalmologists are persuaded to undertake cataract operations.

   (v) Eye banks are being set up.

  (vi) Proper sanitation, safe water supply, health education regarding personal hygiene and care of eyes is being provided.

4. CARDIO-VASCULAR DISEASES

Cardio-vascular diseases are considered as diseases of modern era and are the major cause of death in most of the developed countries. The various cardio-vascular diseases are :

   (i) Coronary heart disease (CHD) or ischaemic heart disease.

   (ii) Rheumatic heart disease.

  (iii) Hypertensive heart disease.

  (iv) Syphilitic heart disease.

   (v) Congenital heart disease.

  (vi) Arrhythmias (abnormal heart rate).

 (vii) Atherosclerosis.

(i) Coronary Heart Disease

There are a number of causes of this disease. The incidence is showing increasing trends. The disease is common in the age group of 50-60 years but the persons around 40 years of age are also showing increasing trends. The males are affected more than the females.

Coronary heart diseases are divided into following groups :

(i) Angina pectoris.

(ii) Myocardial infraction.

(iii) Cardiac failure.

(iv) Sudden death.

(v) Arrhythmias (Abnormal heart rate).

Risk Factors for CHD

(i) Heavy smoking and consumption of alcohol.

(ii) Hypertension.

(iii) High level of serum cholesterol.

(iv) Family history of CHD.

(v) Diabetes mellitus.

(vi) Mental stress and strain in life.

(vii) Lack of physical activity.

(viii) Obesity.

Prevention of CHD

Try to avoid and control the above mentioned factors viz. :

(i) Avoid smoking and excessive consumption of alcohol.

(ii) Control obesity and maintain standard weight.

(iii) Restrict intake of salt, sugar and saturated fatty acids i.e. ghee etc. It should be replaced with poly unsaturated fats.

(iv) Increase consumption of vegetables and fresh fruits.

(v) Ensure optimum regular exercise, relaxed way of life and avoid stress and strain of life.

(vi) Control hypertension and diabetes mellitus.

(vii) Cases of CHD and elderly persons should undergo regular medical checkup.

(ii) Hypertension

Hypertension is derived from two words i.e. hyper means 'excessive' and tension means 'pressure' in this case, of blood. Therefore hypertension means high blood pressure. And blood pressure is the force or pressure exerted by the blood on the inside walls of the blood vessels. Blood pressure greater than 140/90 mm of mercury (systolic/diastolic) in an adult is considered abnormal.

Hypertension or high blood pressure is a major health problem affecting about 20% of the adult population in most countries and is one of the major risk factors for death from cardio-vascular diseases.

High blood pressure is often called a silent killer because it directly kills so many people every year yet much of the time these people have no symptoms of the disease. Therefore persons above 40 years of age must get their blood pressure checked regularly. High blood pressure is more common in males than females specially who belong to intellectual classes and higher socio-economic groups. Based on scientific studies it is proved that blood pressure increases progressively with age.

Types of Hypertension

There are two types of hypertension :

(i) Essential hypertension — When the cause of hypertension is unknown it is known as essential hypertension.

(ii) Secondary hypertension — When the cause of hypertension is due to some disorders it is known as secondary hypertension. The causes of secondary hypertension are :

   (a) Renal diseases e.g. acute glomerulonephritis, pyelonephritis etc.

   (b) Endocrine disorders

   (c) Toxaemia of pregnancy.

Atherosclerosis aggravates hypertension and vice versa.

Risk Factors

   (i) Hereditary and familial tendency.

   (ii) Increasing age above 40 years.

   (iii) Obesity.

   (iv) Stress and strain of life.

   (v) High intake of salt.

   (vi) Over eating and consumption of excess amount of saturated fats.

  (vii) Smoking, tobacco chewing and excessive consumption of alcohol.

 (viii) Lack of physical activity.

   (ix) Use of oral contraceptives.

Signs and Symptoms

   (i) Frequent headache.

  (ii) Pounding of heart and shortness of breath after mild exercise.

 (iii) Weakness, dizziness.

 (iv) Occasional pain in the chest and left shoulder.

Complications

Hypertension increases the workload of heart, weakens the walls of blood vessels and accelerates the hardening of the arteries and the formation of fatty, atherosclerotic deposits inside the blood vessels.

Persons suffering from high blood pressure are far more likely than other people to have strokes, heart failure, coronary heart disease, heart attacks, kidney failure, eye problems and blood vessel disorders.

Prevention and Control

Hypertension can be controlled by adopting following measures :

   (i) Reduce intake of salt by not adding salt to their meals at the table and avoiding salty foods like sauces and pickles. Sometimes a low-salt diet works so well that antihypertensive drugs are not needed or can be greatly reduced.

  (ii) Avoid smoking, chewing of tobacco and excessive consumption of alcohol.

 (iii) Restrict intake of saturated fats in the diet.

 (iv) Reduce weight and do regular physical exercise.

  (v) Avoid stress and strain of life and avoid worries.

 (vi) If high blood pressure is due to kidney disease or some other identifiable cause get it treated at the earliest.

(vii) Use antihypertensive drugs as suggested by the doctor. Such drugs include atenolol, nifedipine, clonidine or alphamethyl dopa. Patients sometimes need a combination of two or three drugs and often must continue taking them for the rest of their lives.

Studies have shown that people whose blood pressure is controlled are far less likely to suffer from cardio-vascular diseases than those whose blood pressure is not controlled.

(iii) Rheumatic Heart Disease (RHD)

Rheumatic heart disease is quite common in India and individuals below 20 years of age suffer from it. Rheumatic fever is a disease of connective tissues particularly in the heart and joints. It is caused by infection of throat by group A beta haemolytic streptococci. It is not a communicable disease but leads to rheumatic heart disease which damages the heart and is a common cause of premature death. High incidence of this disease is due to poverty, undernutrition, overcrowding, poor sanitary conditions and lack of medical facilities.

Clinical Features

Clinical features include fever, inflammation of joints, carditis, subcutaneous nodules, raised ESR and presence of beta haemolytic streptococci in blood culture. The chief organs affected are joints, heart and brain. Brain involvement can lead to tremors.

Prevention and Control

(i) Treat cases of sore throat in children promptly with penicillin. Those having tendency of frequent sore throat should be treated by giving intramuscular injection of crystalline penicillin, procaine penicillin and benzathine penicillin.

(ii) Mass screening of children for rheumatic heart disease should be done through school health services.

(iii) Socio-economic and living conditions of the public should be improved.

(iv) Health education and personal hygiene should be imparted which will be helpful in prevention of the disease.

9

EPIDEMIOLOGY

The word epidemiology is derived from the Greek words, epi means among, demos means people and logos means study. That means it is the study of the distribution of a disease or such a condition in a community. The community may be a village, a city, a country or the whole world. Epidemiology is also derived from the word epidemic.

There are a number of definitions of epidemiology described by different authors but the most suitable definition is that epidemiology may be defined as the detailed scientific study of the distribution and determinants of disease or disability in society. These studies cover sources and modes of transmission of an infection occuring endemically or erupting as an epidemic in the community. It also covers the social, economic and environmental factors.

Earlier the term epidemiology was referred to only those communicable diseases which used to spread in epidemic form like small-pox, cholera, plague etc. but now a days epidemiological studies include communicable, non-communicable, nutritional and deficiency diseases.

USES OF EPIDEMIOLOGY

Following are the major uses of epidemiology :

    (i) To study the history of disease in relation to its rise and fall in a community.

    (ii) To study the respective role of agent, host and environmental factors in the spread of disease.

(iii) It helps in the study of types of diseases prevalent in a community.

(iv) It helps to diagnose the health problems of the community by studying occurrence, distribution by age, sex, occupation and locality.

(v) It helps to find out the morbidity and mortality rates and to identify those individuals or groups at risk or those in need of health care.

(vi) It helps to collect variety of data from different sources which will establish logical chains to explain multiple factors in the spread of a disease.

(vii) It helps to establish epidemiological diagnosis of a disease with better understanding of its different aspects after observing its behaviour in a group of persons. Thus effective preventive and control measures can be adopted.

(viii) It helps in research and experimental studies in the field of medical science.

(ix) It helps to forecast the future trends of the disease which will help to take preventive measures e.g. increased incidence of cholera in summer season and malaria during rainy season.

Though the communicable diseases have been controlled in the developed countries but the non-communicable diseases are on the increase. In under developed or developing countries both communicable and non-communicable diseases are increasing. With the fast urbanisation and industrialisation there is an increased trend in the cases of various malignancies, cardio-vascular diseases, mental and psychosomatic problems, occupational and industrial hazards, accidents etc. In such cases epidemiological studies are carried out on the basis of which preventive and remedial measures are worked out to lessen the intensities of these problems. So the ultimate and final goal of epidemiologists is to study various aspects of diseases and suggest measures for the eradication of the diseases and other problems as far as it is practicable, so as to lessen the sufferings of mankind.

Factors Responsible for the Spread of Communicable Diseases

There are three factors which are responsible for the spread of a disease. These factors include (a) agent (b) host, and (c) environment.

These three factors are known as epidemiological triad. If any one of these three factors is missing then disease cannot occur. These factors are described below :

(a) Agent

Agent is the most important factor for the occurrence of disease. The disease agents include :

  (i) Biological agents like bacteria, viruses, fungi, protozoa, worms and insects.

 (ii) Nutrient agents like carbohydrates, proteins, fats, vitamins, minerals and water. An excess or deficiency of these nutrients may cause nutritional diseases.

(iii) Physical agents like extremes of cold and heat, X-ray, γ-rays, pressure, electricity etc.

(iv) Chemical agents like carbon monoxide, pesticides, fertilizers, fumes, dust, gases etc. may cause illness by inhalation, ingestion or direct contact.

 (v) Mechanical agents like motor vehicles, machinery etc. may cause injuries and fractures.

(b) Host

Man acts as a host to a number of pathogenic micro-organisms. These micro-organisms attack the host when the immunity (i.e. the defence mechanism) is lost. The host related factors include age, sex, heredity, nutrition, occupation, customs and habits etc.

Certain diseases like measles etc. are more common in childhood, cancer in middle age and tuberculosis in old age. Females are more affected from cancer of various organs than males. Cases of heart attacks are more in males than in females. Essential hypertension, diabetes, mental diseases are due to genetic factors. Deficiency of proteins may cause kwashiorkor and other problems. Over-eating may lead to obesity and diabetes. Certain habits like smoking may cause lung cancer, open air defecation may cause soil and water pollution which ultimately causes various types of intestinal disorders.

(c) Environment

Environment plays a great role for the upkeep of health. A healthy environment is crucial for the health and wellbeing of individuals and communities. The environment may be favourable to host or to agent. If the environment is favourable to agent it will cause disease. Climatic and seasonal factors may determine whether it will be suitable to a particular disease or not e.g. malaria is more common in rainy season whereas common cold is more common in winter. Sanitary conditions, provision of potable water supply, education and standard of living as well as biological environment e.g. animals, insects, rodents etc. are important factors in determining incidence of diseases.

Common Terms used in Epidemiology

1. **Infection :** The entry and development or multiplication of a disease producing agent in or on the body of man or animal is known as infection. An infection may or may not lead to a disease state.

2. **Incubation Period :** It is the time interval between the entry of the disease agent into the body of the host and the appearance of the first signs and symptoms of the disease.

3. **Infectious Agent :** Any agent which is capable of producing an infection under favourable conditions of host and environment having the capacity to produce an infectious disease is known as infectious agent.

4. **Infestation :** The lodging, development and reproduction of disease producing agent on the surface of the body or in the intestines is known as infestation.

5. **Incidence :** It signifies the number of persons suffering from a disease during certain prescribed period and is expressed as number of cases per one lac population per year.

6. **Isolation :** It is the complete separation of person or persons suffering from communicable disease from contact with other human beings for the period of communicability.

7. **Contact :** Any person who has remained in association with the infected person or the infected articles can also develop the disease.

8. **Contamination :** It is the presence of infectious agent in or upon the surface of articles, wounds or on inanimate objects such as clothes, food articles, water, toys, utensils, beds, floor etc.

9. **Contagious Disease :** A disease which is transmitted by contact e.g. scabies, trachoma etc. is known as contagious disease.

10. **Communicable Disease :** A disease which is transmitted from one person to another either directly or indirectly through an infectious agent like food, air, water, dust, fomites or contact is known as communicable disease.

11. **Epidemic :** Sudden outbreak of infectious disease that spreads rapidly through the population, affecting a large number of persons in a short period of time is known as epidemic.

12. **Endemic :** When an infectious disease is more or less prevalent in a locality or community it is known as endemic.

13. **Fomites :** Fomites are the inanimate articles other than food or water contaminated by the infectious discharges from a patient and are capable of transmitting the infectious agent to a healthy person. Examples include clothes, towel, handkerchief, pen, pencil, toys, utensils etc.

14. **Host :** A man or animal including birds and arthropods which allows lodgement and development of an infectious agent in its body is known as host. An intermediate host is one in which asexual part of life cycle of the parasite takes place. Definite host is one in which sexual part of life cycle of the parasite takes place.

15. **Non-communicable Diseases :** These are the diseases which are not communicated from person to person but they occur within the patient himself. Examples of such diseases include hypertension, diabetes, blindness, cancer and cardio-vascular diseases.

16. **Notification :** It is the procedure of reporting by earliest and quickest possible time about the occurrence of notifiable disease to the health authorities in order that speedy control and preventive action may be undertaken if necessary. Notifiable diseases may include cholera, diarrhoea, dysentery, infective jaundice, malaria, measles, poliomyelitis, tuberculosis, typhoid and whooping cough.

17. **Pandemic :** When an epidemic spreads from one country to another or even the whole world affecting most of the population then the condition is known as pandemic e.g. AIDS, influenza, cholera and plague pandemics.

18. **Sporadic :** When a disease occurs at intervals and in single,

scattered or isolated cases, it is known as sporadic. Sometimes a sporadic case may be the beginning of an epidemic.

Disease Transmission

All communicable diseases are transmitted from one person to another through some transmission method and they spread from the source or reservoir of infection to a susceptible host. The source of infection may be a person, animal, object or substance from which an infectious agent passes or transmitted to the host. A reservoir may be any person, animal, arthropod, plant, substance or soil (or a combination of these) in which an infectious agent lives and multiplies from where it can be transmitted to the susceptible host. For example reservoir for tetanus bacilli is the soil but the host is man. Similarly reservoir for rabies virus is an animal but the host may be animal or man.

For planning suitable prevention and control measures it is essential to know the manner in which the diseases are transmitted which are discussed below.

Routes or Channels of Infection

Following are the routes by which the infection enters the body :

(i) Through skin and mucous membrane — Some organisms may enter the body through the skin or mucous membrane. For example malaria is spread by biting of mosquitoes and rabies is spread by biting of rabid animals. Syphilis, gonorrhoea and AIDS is spread through mucous membrane.

(ii) Through respiratory tract — Inhalation of air carrying various micro-organisms are responsible for a number of infectious diseases e.g. pulmonary tuberculosis, diphtheria, influenza etc.

(iii) Through gastro-intestinal tract — Ingestion of infected food or drinks may cause infection through gastro-intestinal tract e.g. diarrhoea, cholera, enteric fever etc.

Modes of Transmission of Infection

Infection may be transmitted from the reservoir to the host by the following modes :

A. **Direct transmission**

(a) Direct contact

(b) Droplet infection

(c) Infected dust

(d) Animal bite

(e) Transplacental transmission

B. **Indirect Transmission**

(a) Vehicle borne

(b) Vector borne

(c) Fomite borne.

A. Direct Transmission

In direct transmission infection is spread without any intermediate host.

(a) **Direct Contact :** Some diseases are spread from person to person by direct contact e.g. shaking hands, kissing, sexual contact etc. Diseases spread by direct contact include diarrhoea, dysentery, cholera, typhoid, syphilis, gonorrhoea and AIDS.

(b) **Droplet Infection :** When a person with respiratory infection coughs, sneezes or talks loudly, fine droplets are thrown out which contain large number of pathogenic micro-organisms. When these droplets are inhaled by healthy persons, they also get infected. This type of infection is known as droplet infection which is the most common mode of transmission of diseases. Diseases spread by droplet infection include common cold, influenza, tuberculosis, measles, whooping cough, smallpox, chickenpox, diphtheria, viral and pneumococcal pneumonia etc.

(c) **Infected Dust :** Some of the droplets containing pathogenic micro-organisms which are expelled during talking, laughing, coughing or sneezing by the diseased person either settle down on articles like clothes, bedding, carpets or on floor and other objects. These droplets dry up over there and during dusting, bed making and sweeping, the dust is released into the air which if inhaled by the healthy persons will infect them. Dust particles may also be blown by wind from soil. The diseases which are caused by infected dust include enteric fever, cholera, amoebic dysentery, pneumonia, tuberculosis and tetanus.

(d) **Animal Bite :** Some infections occur due to animal bite e.g. dog bite, snake bite etc.

(e) **Transplacental Transmission :** Some disease agents may be transmitted from the infected mother to the foetus through the placenta. This kind of transmission is known as vertical transmission. Examples include hepatitis B, rubella virus, syphilis and AIDS etc.

B. Indirect Transmission

When the disease agent is transmitted from diseased person to healthy person through some substance like milk, water, insects or fomites it is known· as indirect transmission.

(a) **Vehicle Borne :** The common vehicles through which disease agent is transmitted include water, milk, food, blood, blood products, tissues and organs. The diseases which are spread through water, food or blood are known as water borne, food borne or blood borne diseases respectively. Water borne and food borne diseases are the most common ones which include infections of the alimentary tract such as enteric fever, cholera, diarrhoea, dysentery, hepatitis A, food poisoning etc. Milk borne diseases are also quite important because milk is a good culture medium for bacteria and easily gets infected. When infected milk is consumed by the healthy persons they also get the infection. The diseases spread by infected milk include bovine tuberculosis, diphtheria, sore throat, enteric fever and dysentery. The most important disease transmitted through infected blood is hepatitis B (serum hepatitis).

(b) **Vector Borne :** A vector may be defined as an arthropod or any living organism that transfers the infectious agent to the susceptible host. Examples of such arthropods include mosquito (malaria), rat flea (plague), louse (typhus fever), flies etc. Vector borne trans-mission may be simply mechanical as the house flies carry the disease agent from one place to another on their body, wings and legs. Mosquito acts as an intermediate host in malaria and filariasis where sexual part of malarial parasite develops in the body of the mosquito. The vector borne diseases include malaria, filaria, kala-azar and plague etc.

(c) **Fomite Borne :** Fomites are the inanimate articles which are capable of absorbing, retaining or transferring infection from one person to another. The articles which come in direct contact with the patient easily get contaminated with disease agent and can spread disease to the healthy persons when they come in contact with such articles. Examples of fomites are clothes, towels, handkerchief, bedding, spoons, drinking glasses, utensils, pen, pencil, books, removed dressings, toys etc. Such articles contaminated with pathogenic micro-organisms play an important role in the indirect transmission of infections.

General Methods of Prevention and Control of Communicable Diseases

As discussed earlier three components i.e. agent, mode of transmission and host are very important for the spread of a disease. If any of these components is missing then disease cannot spread, therefore measures should be taken to control these components so as to prevent the spread of diseases.

A. Controlling the Source of Infection

(i) **Early Diagnosis :** The first and most important point in the control of infectious disease is the early and accurate diagnosis of the disease. If the disease is properly treated at source and disease agent is destroyed then the chances of spread of the disease will be minimized.

(ii) **Notification :** Notifiable diseases should be immediately reported to the health authorities who will take proper measures to control the disease.

(iii) **Isolation :** Patients suffering from communicable diseases should be isolated so as to limit the spread of the disease to the public. The period of isolation varies from disease to disease, usually it is as long as the 'infectious' period of the disease. Isolation can be done either in the hospital or at home. Hospital isolation, where possible is always better than home isolation because of restrictions imposed and specialized facilities available in the hospital.

(iv) **Treatment :** If proper treatment is given at an early stage of the disease, it will shorten the duration of the disease and lessen the sufferings of the patient. Early treatment with antibiotics will kill the pathogenic micro-organisms thus the spread of infection will be prevented. Prophylactic and therapeutic treatment can be given.

B. Blocking the Modes of Transmission

Modes of transmission of infection should be controlled by adopting following measures :

    (i) Drinking water should be properly disinfected.

    (ii) All food items should be protected from disease agents.

    (iii) Human excreta should be disposed of in a sanitary way.

    (iv) Overall standard of living should be improved.

    (v) Mosquitoes, flies, other insects, rodents and stray dogs should be destroyed.

    (vi) All discharges of the patient should be disposed of in a sanitary manner.

    (vii) All fomites of the patient should be thoroughly disinfected and disposable items should be burnt.

    (viii) Transmission of sexually transmitted diseases can be prevented by using mechanical contraceptives.

    If above mentioned points are given due consideration then the transmission of diseases can be controlled to a great extent.

C. Protecting the Susceptible Host

  (i) **Immunization :** Some of the diseases like diphtheria, pertusis, tetanus, measles, poliomyelitis, tuberculosis can only be controlled through proper immunization. Immunization is a cheap, safe, effective and easy method for the control of majority of infectious diseases. For certain diseases no effective vaccine is available therefore in such cases other health systems should be used to control the disease e.g. in malaria, diarrhoea, certain respiratory infections etc.

  (ii) **Health Education :** If health education regarding mode of spread and method of prevention of various diseases is imparted to the public then with their active co-operation a large number of communicable diseases can be controlled easily, effectively and within short period of time.

Immunological Preparations

Immunology is the study of immunity and preparations used to produce immunity are called immunological preparations. All immunological preparations are biological products which are administered parenterally to avoid inactivation of the preparation on oral administration. The exception is poliomyelitis vaccine which is administered orally. It contains living viruses which can multiply in the gut.

Immunity

The infection or disease in human beings or animals is caused by the invasion of pathogenic micro-organisms. The power of the body to resist the effects of invasion of pathogenic micro-organisms is known as immunity and lack of power of the body to resist infection is called susceptibility.

There are a number of factors which are responsible for immunity but phagocytosis and antibody formation are most important.

(i) **Phagocytosis :** Phagocytosis may be defined as the ingestion of micro-organisms by certain cells of the body whereby they are rendered harmless. Phagocytosis is caused by (i) white blood corpuscles (WBCs) and the cells of the reticuloendothelial system. The white blood cells freely float in the blood and are carried continuously to all the tissues. When the micro-organisms enter the body, more and more WBCs collect at the site of infection and ingest the invading bacteria, rendering them harmless. The cells of the reticuloendothelial system present in the blood spaces of liver and spleen ingest the micro-organisms when the blood stream passes through liver and spleen and render the micro-organisms harmless which are then carried to lungs where they are disintegrated.

(ii) **Antibody Production :** The body does not depend only on the process of phagocytosis for the destruction of pathogenic micro-organisms. It produces other substances known as antibodies which destroy the pathogenic micro-organisms and their toxins. Antibodies are highly specific in their nature and attack either micro-organisms or toxins.

Antibodies may be defined as the substances produced in the body, on the invasion of pathogenic micro-organisms either to destory these pathogenic micro-organisms or their toxins.

Types of Immunity

Immunity may be classified as follows :

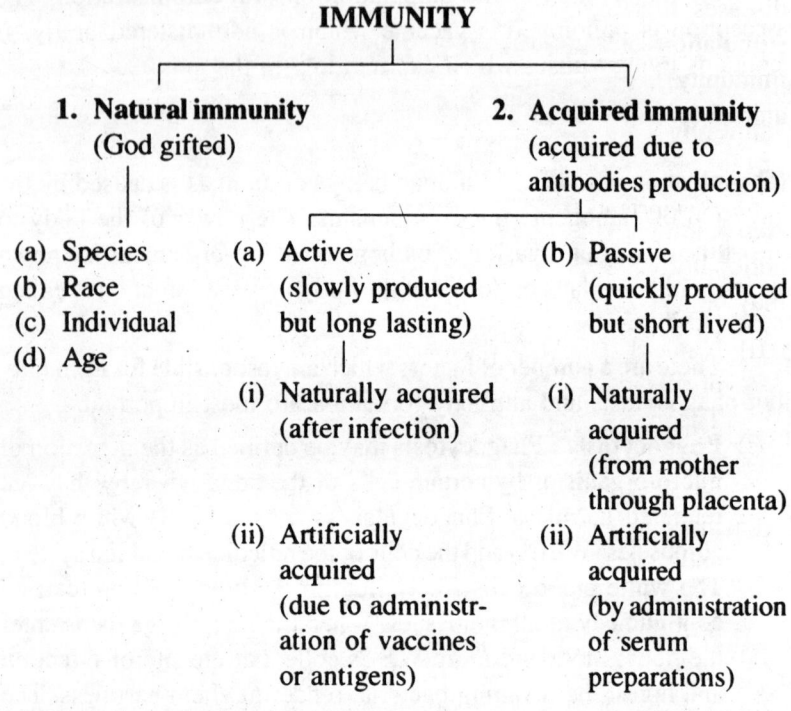

IMMUNITY

1. Natural immunity
(God gifted)

2. Acquired immunity
(acquired due to
antibodies production)

(a) Species
(b) Race
(c) Individual
(d) Age

(a) Active
(slowly produced
but long lasting)

(i) Naturally acquired
(after infection)

(ii) Artificially
acquired
(due to administr-
ation of vaccines
or antigens)

(b) Passive
(quickly produced
but short lived)

(i) Naturally
acquired
(from mother
through placenta)

(ii) Artificially
acquired
(by administration
of serum
preparations)

1. Natural Immunity

It is God gifted immunity which exerts resistance to disease. It differs between species, races, individuals and ages.

(a) **Species :** Certain species are immune to some diseases whereas others are not. For example man is susceptible to plague but fowls are not; tuberculosis is very fatal to guinea-pigs but is not so fatal to man.

(b) **Races :** Negroes have high resistance to yellow fever whereas white men are susceptible to it.

(c) **Individuals :** It is well known that some persons are more resistant to cold and skin infections than others.

(d) **Age :** Most of the children between 2-5 years of age group are susceptible to diphtheria whereas most adults are immune to it.

2. Acquired Immunity

Natural immunity is not sufficient to protect the body from microbial diseases therefore additional immunity is acquired either by the stimulation of the antibody producing cells of the body (active immunity) or by introducing antibodies formed from another person or animal (passive immunity)

(a) Active Immunity

Active immunity is developed in an individual due to the formation of antibodies on the introduction of antigenic substances in the body. It may be naturally acquired or artificially stimulated.

(i) **Naturally Acquired Active Immunity :** It is acquired as a result of natural infection produced by pathogenic micro-organisms. There may or may not be a clinically recognisable disease. When a patient recovers from certain diseases like diphtheria, small-pox, poliomyelitis, he is left with a high degree of immunity which may last for the whole life, however after influenza. pneumonia and gonorrhoea, immunity produced is short lived. Similarly children living in slum areas acquire immunity against a number of diseases because they are exposed to such diseases time and again.

(ii) **Artificially Acquired Active Immunity :** This type of immunity is acquired by the administration of specific vaccines or toxoids. When these antigenic substances are introduced into the body, they stimulate the body to produce antibodies. Thus body develops its own defence against pathogenic micro-organisms.

(b) Passive Immunity

This type of immunity is produced by the introduction of already formed antibodies into the body of an individual. These antibodies may have been developed in another individual or even in another species. Though passive immunity is rapidly produced but it is not long lasting. Passive immunity may be naturally acquired or artificially produced.

(i) **Naturally Acquired Passive Immunity :** In this type of immunity the antibodies are transmitted from the mother to the foetus through the placental blood. This imparts immunity to the infant for several months. Antibodies for chickenpox, diphtheria, measles and scarlet fever are transmitted in this way, that is why the infants show high resistance against these diseases only for about six months after which this resistance is lost.

(ii) **Artificially Produced Passive Immunity :** This type of immunity is produced by injecting antibodies-containing preparations known as antisera, sera or immune sera. The antibodies are first produced in an animal usually a horse or occasionally some other person and then injected into the concerned person.

Related Terms Used in Immunity

1. **Pathogens :** These are the infection causing micro-organisms.

2. **Antigens :** These are the substances which stimulate the body to produce antibodies.

3. **Antibodies :** These are the substances formed in the body in response to stimulation by antigens.

4. **Toxins :** These are the poisonous substances produced by pathogenic micro-organisms and lead to infection or disease in man or animals.

5. **Exotoxins :** These are the toxins which can diffuse freely through the bacterial cell wall into the blood of the medium in which the micro-organisms are growing.

6. **Endotoxins :** These are the toxins which cannot diffuse through the bacterial cell wall and are retained within the bacteria. They are released only when the cells die and start disintegrating.

7. **Antitoxins :** These are the substances containing antibodies produced by the blood, which specifically neutralise the toxins produced by particular micro-organisms.

8. **Sera or immune sera :** A clear fluid which separates from blood when it clots is known as serum. When a serum contains antitoxic antibodies it is known as antitoxic serum. They are usually obtained from animals but sometimes from human serum also.

9. **Toxoids :** These are the toxins whose toxicity has been removed by gentle heat or by chemical treatment but their antigenic

properties are retained e.g. tetanus toxoid and staphylococcus toxoid.

10. **Vaccines :** These are the substances which are administered in the body to produce resistance against infectious diseases. They are mainly used as prophylactic treatment. Vaccines may contain living, attenuated or killed bacteria, viruses or rickettsia.

Forms of Vaccines

(i) **Simple Vaccines :** These vaccines contain only one species of micro-organisms.

(ii) **Mixed Vaccines :** These vaccines contain two or more than two species of micro-organisms.

(iii) **Univalent Vaccines :** These vaccines contain only one strain of a species.

(iv) **Polyvalent Vaccines :** These vaccines contain two or more strains of the same species of micro-organisms.

IMMUNOLOGICAL PREPARATIONS

These are the substances or agents which are used to produce immunity in an individual. They are mainly used for the prevention of diseases e.g. vaccines. They are also used for the treatment of diseases e.g. antiserums; and also for diagnostic purposes e.g. bacterial toxins.

Classification of Immunological Preparations

The immunological preparations may be classified as follows :

1. Preparations producing active immunity

(a) Vaccines containing living bacteria e.g. B.C.G. vaccine.

(b) Vaccines containing dead bacteria e.g. cholera, pertussis, plague and typhoid vaccine.

(c) Vaccines containing killed rickettesia e.g. typhus vaccine.

(d) Vaccines containing living viruses e.g. measles, small-pox, poliomyelitis and yellow fever.

(e) Vaccines containing toxoids e.g. diphtheria, tetanus and staphylococcus.

2. Diagnostic preparations containing bacterial toxins used for Schick test and tuberculin test.

3. Preparations containing antibodies (antitoxin and antiserum) used to produce passive immunity.

Immunization Schedule

All the pregnant women, infants and children at specified time must be vaccinated against communicable diseases so as to give protection against such diseases which include diphtheria, pertussis, tetanus, polio, tuberculosis and measles. All the countries have their own immunization schedule which is based on their local needs and feasibility. This schedule may vary from region to region. While deciding immunization schedule following points must be taken into consideration :

  (i) Age of the child

 (ii) Availability of effective vaccines

(iii) Cost of the vaccine

(iv) Minimum number of visits to the health centre by the mother and the child.

National immunization schedule is given in the following table (Table 9.1).

A programme named Expanded Programme of Immunization (EPI) was started by WHO in the year 1974 throughout the world. According to this programme it was proposed to immunize all children by 1990 against six diseases viz., diphtheria, pertussis, tetanus, polio, tuberculosis, and measles. But in the year 1990 the name of this programme was changed to Universal Child Immunization (UCI - 1990). According to this programme every child must be immunized in the first year of age.

Hospital-Acquired Infection

Hospital-acquired infections are also known as nosocomial infections. They are defined as the infections acquired by the patient after they have been admitted to the hospital or other health care centre. Prior to admission in the hospital the patients do not have any such disease. They can get the disease from different sources like patients, unsterilised instruments, infected hands of surgeons, nurses, ward boys and other hospital staff who come in contact with the patients. Contaminated food, water and other drinks may also be a good source of infection. Articles like linen, bed clothes, furniture, sinks, basins,

Table 9.1 : National Immunization Schedule

Beneficiaries	Age group	Name of vaccine	No of doses	Route of administration	Remarks
Pregnant women	16 to 36 weeks	Tetanus toxoid (T.T.)	1	Intramuscular	Two doses if not vaccinated previously.
Infants	6 weeks to 9 months	DPT Polio oral polio vaccine (OPV)	3 3	Intramuscular Oral	Each dose is given at an interval of one month. Each dose is given at an interval of one month.
		BCG	1	Intradermal	In hospital deliveries BCG vaccine should be given at birth.
	9 to 12 months	Measles	1	Subcutaneous	
Children	16 to 24 months	DPT (booster dose) OPV (booster dose)	1 1	Intramuscular Oral	

(Contd.)

Beneficiaries	Age group	Name of vaccine	No of doses	Route of administration	Remarks
	5 to 6 years	DT	1	Intramuscular	Two doses, if not vaccinated previously
		Typhoid	2	Subcutaneous	At an interval of one month.
	10 years	Tetanus toxoid (T.T.)	1	Intramuscular	Two doses, if not vaccinated previously.
		Typhoid	1	Subcutaneous	Two doses, if not vaccinated previously.
	16 years	Tetanus toxoid (T.T.)	1	Intramuscular	Two doses, if not vaccinated earlier.
		Typhoid	1	Subcutaneous	Two doses, if not vaccinated previously.

National immunisation schedule is followed throughout the country.

pots, door handles etc. are also a source of infection. Hospital dust, air and discharges of the patient which are highly contaminated with micro-organisms, are the most important sources of infection.

Hospital acquired infections include cross infections i.e. infection from person to person and autoinfections i.e. infections from one tissue to another tissue in the same patient e.g. discharging wounds, infected skin lesions, eczema, psoriasis, boils, bed sores etc.

The common pathogenic micro-organisms responsible for hospital acquired infection include staphylococcus, streptococcus, E. coli, corynebacterium diptheriae, clostridium tetani, hepatitis virus through infected blood. etc.

The common hospital acquired infections include infections of alimentary tract, infections of respiratory tract, infections of urinary tract, wound infections, skin infections, viral infections etc.

Prevention and Control

Hospital acquired infections can be prevented by adopting following measures :

(i) Isolate the infectious patient.

(ii) Doctors, nurses and other staff attending the patient must take precautions for personal hygiene. They should wear face mask and apron. They must wash the hands with soap and water after attending each infected patient specially after doing the wound dressings. Sometimes hand washing with soap and water may not be sufficient so a disinfectant must be used for hand washing.

(iii) The articles used by the patient should be thoroughly disinfected.

(iv) Wound dressings and discharges of the patient like urine, faeces, nasal secretions, sputum etc. should be destroyed in a sanitary manner.

(v) Patients should not be allowed to spit here and there. They should spit only in the sputum cup containing some disinfectant.

(vi) There should be sufficient space in between the beds of two patients. The bed side pans must contain some disinfectant and they must be cleaned immediately after use.

(vii) Vacuum cleaning and wet cleaning of rooms should be done regularly and disinfectant used to kill the micro-organisms.

(viii) Rooms should be well-ventilated, all doors and windows should be fitted with wire gauge to prevent the entry of flies, mosquitoes and other insects in the rooms.

(ix) All instruments, needles and syringes used should be properly sterilized, preferably disposable needles and syringes should be used.

(x) Staff working in the kitchen must observe strict hygienic habits and must be periodically medically examined so as to ensure that they are free from infectious diseases.

(xi) Laboratory personnel handling various specimens should observe all precautions to prevent infections.

(xii) Entry of visitors should be restricted in the rooms where patients with communicable diseases are admitted.

(xiii) Patients suffering from communicable diseases should be properly treated with antibiotics and measures should be taken to avoid the spread of the disease to other patients.

DISINFECTION

Various common terms used are :

(i) Disinfection

Disinfection is the process of killing the pathogenic microorganisms from the inanimate articles.

(ii) Disinfectants

Disinfectants are the agents which are used to kill the pathogenic microorganisms which cause communicable diseases. Such substances include chemical and physical agents. They are too corrosive or toxic that they cannot be applied on the living tissues so they are used on inanimate surfaces.

(iii) Deodorant

A deodorant is a substance which is used to suppress bad odour e.g. lime, bleaching powder.

(iv) Detergent

A detergent is a chemical agent which is used to clean the surfaces by lowering surface tension e.g. soap is used to remove bacteria, dirt and oily materials from surfaces.

(v) Antiseptics

Antiseptics are the agents which are used to kill or inhibit the growth of infectious agents. These can be applied to living tissues e.g. alcohol, dettol etc. A disinfectant in low concentrations or dilutions can be used as an antiseptic.

(vi) Insecticides

These are the agents used to kill insects e.g. D.D.T.

(vii) Repellants

These are the agents used to repel the insects e.g. Odomos etc.

(viii) Sterilization

Sterilization is the process of complete destruction of bacteria and spores by different methods like physical, chemical, ionisation and gaseous sterilization. In hospitals it is not possible to do sterilization for each and every article so in routine, disinfection is done which is the most popular method of destroying the pathogenic microorganisms from inanimate articles.

TYPES OF DISINFECTION

Disinfection is classified into three categories :

    (i) Concurrent disinfection
    (ii) Terminal disinfection
    (iii) Prophylactic disinfection

(i) Concurrent Disinfection

Concurrent disinfection means immediate destruction of infectious material excreted by the patient like faeces, urine, sputum and vomitings. Soiled clothes, bed sheets, dressings etc. are also immediately disinfected as soon as they are soiled with the discharges of the patient.

(ii) Terminal Disinfection

In terminal disinfection, along with the concurrent disinfection when the patient is discharged or dies all his beddings, utensils, furniture and room is disinfected so as to prevent the transmission of infection to other patients.

(iii) Prophylactic Disinfection

Washing of hands with soap and water, boiling of water, pasteurization of milk and treatment of tap water with chlorine are some of the examples of prophylactic disinfectants.

CLASSIFICATION OF DISINFECTANTS

Disinfectants are classified as follows :

    (a) Natural e.g. air and sunlight

    (b) Physical e.g. burning, dry heat, boiling, steam under pressure, radiations.

    (c) Chemical e.g. liquids, solids and gaseous.

(A) NATURAL DISINFECTANTS

Fresh air and sunlight act as natural disinfectants because air dries up the moisture present in bacteria which is lethal to bacteria. Air also takes away the infectious material which gets diluted in large volume of the air and becomes less harmful.

Direct and continuous exposure to sunlight is very harmful to bacteria due to the presence of ultraviolet rays in sunlight. Beddings and furniture may be exposed to strong sunlight for several hours for terminal disinfection.

(B) PHYSICAL DISINFECTANTS

(i) Burning

Burning is a very good and cheap method of disinfection. Inexpensive materials like dressings, swabs and rags can be disposed of by burning.

But burning of infectious materials should be done in a specially designed apparatus known as incinerator. If incinerator is not available then burning should be done in the open away from the habitation. For burning the wet dressings etc. some saw dust and kerosene oil may be put on the materials and then burnt.

(ii) Dry Heat

Dry heat has a very low penetrating power, so bacterial spores are not easily killed by this method. Therefore a high temperature has to be maintained for a long time. For this purpose hot air oven is used where a temperature of 160° to 180°C is maintained.

Dry heat is not suitable for heavy articles like mattresses etc. moreover it destroys nearly all fabrics. This method is used for disinfection of glassware, syringes, swabs, dressings and sharp instruments.

(iii) Boiling

Boiling is a cheap and efficient method of disinfection. Boiling the material in water for 15-20 minutes kills all germs and boiling for 30 minutes may kill all spores. This method is quite suitable for linen, handkerchiefs, bed sheets, cooking utensils, syringes etc. For disinfecting the syringes, the plunger and the body of the syringe should be separated, wraped in gauge and then boiled in water. Germicidal power of boiling water is increased if 1% soap and washing soda is added to boiling water specially it is useful for disinfecting the linen and bed sheets etc. The clothes stained with blood or faeces must be washed with cold water first and then boiled in water. Otherwise a permanent stain of blood or faeces will be produced.

Boiling has disadvantages that :

(a) It is a slow process.

(b) It is unsuitable for thick linens.

(c) It is not suitable for woollen and synthetic clothes as they shrink and get destroyed by boiling.

(d) It produces permanent stains of blood and faeces.

(e) Sharp instruments get blunt by boiling.

(iv) Steam Under Pressure

Steam under pressure (saturated steam) is the most effective method of disinfection in hospitals and laboratories. For this purpose an autoclave is used. Steam under pressure can penetrate better than ordinary steam thus sterilization is more effective. When steam under pressure comes in contact with materials to be sterilized it immediately gives away latent heat and sterilizes them. Steam under pressure is the most relable method of disinfection for linen, gloves, dressings, syringes, certain instruments, glass apparatus and culture media. This method should not be used for sterilization of plastics and sharp instruments. The articles which have been sterilized by autoclaving should not be exposed to the environment before use as they may get contaminated.

(v) Ionising Radiations

Sterilization by ionising radiations is a newer technique and is being increasingly used for sterilization of bandages, dressings, surgical instruments and catgut. The agents used for this purpose include :

(a) Infrared rays from electrically heated element.

(b) Ultraviolet rays from sunlight or mercury vapour lamp.

(c) Ionising by isotopes or X-rays.

The materials to be sterilized are put in polythene bags which are then exposed to ionising radiations. These radiations have strong penetrating power with little or no heating effect. The advantages of this method are that :

(i) The materials remain sterile until the bags are opened.

(ii) It is most effective method of sterilization. The disadvantage of this method is that it a very costly method.

(C) CHEMICAL DISINFECTANTS

Articles which cannot be sterilized by heat (dry heat or moist heat) may be sterilized by chemical agents. The manner in which the chemical disinfectants act is not fully understood. They chiefly act by oxidising and coagulating the protoplasm of bacteria. They also act by ionic coagulation, dessication, emulsoid action, absorption etc.

Various types of chemical disinfectants include :

(a) Liquids e.g. phenol, lysol, hexachlorophane, chlorhexidine

(hibitane) chloroxylenol (dettol), cetrimide, savlon, iodine, chlorine, hydrogen peroxide, alcohol, methylated spirit, formalin, acetone, mercurochrome, gentian violet, acriflavin etc.

(b) Solids e.g. lime, bleaching powder, DDT, BHC, potassium permanganate, mercuric iodide etc.

(c) Gaseous e.g. chlorine, ethylene oxide, formalin, sulphur dioxide and hydrocyanic acid gas etc.

DISINFECTION PROCEDURES

(i) Faeces and Urine

Faeces and urine should be collected in an impervious container to which an equal volume of 8% bleaching powder, 10% formalin solution, 5% cresol or 10% phenol is added. The disinfectant is allowed to remain in contact for at least two hours. After disinfection the container is emptied in a drain.

If more of the above mentioned chemical is available then boiling water is put in the container and allowed to remain in contact till it cools down. Alternatively the stools are emptied in a drain or buried and covered with lime.

(ii) Sputum

On small scale the sputum is collected in paper containers or on handkerchief which is burnt immediately after collecting the sputum. When the quantity of sputum excreted is large as in the case of T.B. then it is collected either in disposable paper cups or in sputum cups half filled with cresol solution. The patient should spit in these cups and when full they are allowed to stand for two hours and then disposed of. Alternatively a large amount of sputum can be disinfected by boiling or autoclaving for 20 minutes at 20 pounds pressure and then disposed of.

(iii) Room

The walls of hospital rooms and operation theatres are generally painted with washable paints and floors are made of chips or marble which can be easily cleaned by washing with water. Generally the rooms which are well ventilated and direct sunlight enters into the

rooms, do not require any disinfection but if need arises then floor and walls are mopped with soap or any detergent then washed with good flow of water. No body should be allowed to enter in the room for the next two days.

Chemical disinfection can be carried out by using 2 to 3% cresol, 5% phenol, 10% formalin solution or a concentrated solution of bleaching powder. The floor and walls of the room are mopped with any of the above mentioned solutions which is allowed to remain in contact for 4 to 6 hours then it is washed with free flow of water.

For operation theatres above mentioned treatment is carried out. After this the theatre is fumigated with gaseous formaldehyde. For this purpose 500 ml of formalin is mixed with one litre of water, the solution is boiled and the fumes are generated. The room so treated is kept closed for 12 hours and then it can be used.

(iv) Linen

Linen, bed sheets and other clothings should be disinfected by boiling in water for half to one hour. If soap is added to water the disinfectant action is enhanced. Linen soiled with excreta, pus or blood should be first soaked in 10% formalin or 5% phenol solution. Then they are boiled in soap and water for about two hours.

Woollen articles, leather goods and furniture etc. cannot be disinfected by boiling or autoclaving. Such articles should be disinfected by ionising radiations.

(v) Instruments

Syringes, needles, glass articles of routine use are disinfected by boiling in water for 20-30 minutes. The articles which get spoiled by boiling should be disinfected by ionising radiations. Boiling does not kill the spores so surgical instruments cannot be sterilized by boiling, they should be autoclaved. Very sharp and sophisticated instruments, rubber articles should be disinfected by ionising radiations.

(vi) Dead bodies

The disposal of dead bodies is not new. Some system was adopted for their disposal from time immemorial. It is carried out in different systems in different communities. In India three systems are adopted namely burning, burying and floating the body in water.

Burning of the dead body is a unique method which is adopted by many communities. By burning the body of diseased person all the pathogenic microorganisms are killed. While taking the dead body of the diseased person it must be covered with a cloth soaked in disinfectant so as to prevent the chances of infection pouring out of the body.

In big cities like Calcutta, Madras, Bombay, Delhi etc. the dead bodies are disposed of by burning the body in high currents of heat provided by electric furnace. By this method the body is reduced to ashes within half an hour.

In burying the dead bodies are buried under deep earth. It is also a good method of disposal of dead bodies but not as good as burning. The Mohammedans and Christians adopt this method. The main disadvantage of burying is that it requires lot of land.

The third method of disposal of dead bodies is to float the dead body in a nearby river, stream or sea. This system is not the right method of disposing of dead bodies because once it is floated in water, it is eaten up by the water animals. Though it is an easy method of disposal of dead bodies but it is improper method because it pollutes, contaminates and creates unhygienic conditions and water becomes unfit for human consumption.

INDEX